Your *Own* Pharmacy

The guide for GPs

David Roberts

Application – patient survey
– legal advice
? no more applications for 5 years?

Radcliffe Publishing
Oxford • San Francisco

Radcliffe Publishing Ltd
18 Marcham Road
Abingdon
Oxon OX14 1AA
United Kingdom

www.radcliffe-oxford.com
Electronic catalogue and worldwide online ordering facility.

British Library Cataloguing in Publication Data

A catalogue record for this book is available from the British Library.

ISBN 1 85775 630 4

Typeset by Aarontype Ltd, Easton, Bristol
Printed and bound by TJ International Ltd, Padstow, Cornwall

Contents

Preface

This book is primarily for general medical practitioners and especially those who may both want, and be able to, take the step of opening their own pharmacy within their own premises. There may shortly be regulation changes that could make that step easier for a considerable number of doctors working in so-called one-stop health care centres.

There will also be a large number of doctors who have never given the subject a moment's thought, but who, on reading through the book, may well find that they too, could own a pharmacy, even under the present regulations. Hopefully all the information they will need to tempt them to take the step is within these pages.

A third group of readers are the general practitioners (GPs) who really have no idea what goes on behind the scenes in the high-street chemist's shop. When they put the book down they will be enlightened and may even look at their fellow professionals through new eyes.

Dispensing doctors form another group who may have an interest in how a pharmacy is run and the responsibilities of pharmacists. They are close to my heart and I hope that they too are able to get something out of the book.

The final group who may find something of interest here are the pharmacy students who have yet to decide which branch of his profession to follow. Whilst I make no pretence that the 200 pages of *Your Own Pharmacy* is a comprehensive textbook on community pharmacy, it does, I hope, give more than an idea of what would be in store (excuse the pun) for the student who goes on to choose the community rather than the hospital.

There is a word of caution here. The New Pharmacy Contract was under deep discussion whilst the book was being prepared. It may make community pharmacy even more attractive — who knows — but it will certainly change it.

As every author says at this stage, all the errors and omissions are mine and mine alone and I accept complete responsibility for them. I would be delighted if any glaringly obvious errors that I may have made could be relayed to me through the publisher.

Finally, I would like to thank all those background helpers who have advised me throughout the preparation of the book. Not least among those are the very many proofreaders, project managers and other unsung heroes at Radcliffe Publishing and elsewhere. To all of you, a large thank you.

David Roberts
August 2004

About the author

David Roberts has been a rural dispensing doctor for his entire career since qualifying in 1967, first in Hertfordshire and for 25 years in Husbands Bosworth, Leicestershire. In 1984, he entered medical politics by founding the original Dispensing Doctors Association and in the early 1990s he was elected to the Council of the British Medical Association, a seat he holds at the time of writing. Throughout his career David Roberts has maintained a very keen interest in doctor dispensing and pharmacy, producing four editions of *The Complete Dispenser* – still the only textbook on dispensing practice. *Your Own Pharmacy* complements that book. He is now in a state of semi-retirement.

List of abbreviations

ACAS	Arbitration, Conciliation, and Arbitration Service
A&E	accident and emergency
AGM	annual general meeting
APPS	Association of Professional Pharmacy Staff
APT	Association of Pharmacy Technicians
BMA	British Medical Association
BMI	body-mass index
BNF	*British National Formulary*
BRC	British Retail Consortium
BS	British Standards
C&E	Customs & Excise
CCTV	closed-circuit television
CD	controlled or dangerous drug
CDA	Chemists Defence Association
CHC	Community Health Council
CHRE	Council for Healthcare Regulatory Excellence
CPA	Consumer Protection Act
CPD	continuing professional development
CPO	crime prevention officer
CRE	Commission for Racial Equality
CRHP	Commission for the Regulation of Healthcare Professions
DDA	Disability Discrimination Act
DDA	Dispensing Doctors Association
DoH	Department of Health
EHR	electronic health record
EPOS	electronic point of sale
ESPS	Essential Small Pharmacy Scheme
ETP	electronic transmission of prescription
EU	European Union
FPO	fire prevention officer
GMC	General Medical Council
GMS	General Medical Services
GMSC	General Medical Services Committee
GPC	General Practitioners Committee
GSL	general sales list
HA	health authority
INR	international normalised ratio
IPM	Institute of Pharmacy Management
IR	Inland Revenue
IT	Industrial Tribunal
LA	local authority

LIFT	Local Improvement and Finance Trust
LMC	local medical committee
LPC	local pharmaceutical committee
MDS	monitored dosage system
MDU	Medical Defence Union
MIMS	Monthly Index of Medical Specialities
MMS	Medicines Management Services
MPharm	Master of Pharmacy
NACOSS	National Approved Council for Security Systems
NHS	National Health Service
NPA	National Pharmaceutical Association
NPSA	National Patient Safety Agency
NSF	National Service Framework
OFT	Office of Fair Trading
OS	operating system
OTC	over the counter
P	pharmacy (on non-prescription medicine)
P-only	prescription-only medicine
PACT	Prescribing Analysis and CosT data
PAGB	Proprietary Association of Great Britain
PC	politically correct
PCO	primary care organisation
PCPA	Primary Care Pharmacists Association
PCT	primary care trust
PDA	Pharmacists Defence Association
PL	product licence
PMIC	Pharmacy Mutual Insurance Company
PMR	patient medication record
POM	prescription only medicine
PPA	Prescription Pricing Authority
PPRB	Prescription Price Regulation Board
PREM	premises
PS	Pharmaceutical Society
PSNC	Pharmaceutical Services Negotiating Committee
R&D	research and development
RPA	Rural Pharmacists Association
RPM	retail price maintenance
RPS	Royal Pharmaceutical Society
RPSGB	Royal Pharmaceutical Society of Great Britain
SFA	Statement of Fees and Allowances
SHA	strategic health authority
SOP	standard operating procedure
SPF	Scottish Pharmaceutical Federation
SSAIB	Security Systems and Alarms Inspection Board
SSDP	Strategic Service Development Plan
UCA	Ulster Chemists Association
USP	unique selling point
YPG	Young Pharmacists Group
ZD	Zero Discount

Chapter 1

An opportunity created

The very title — *Your Own Pharmacy* — will mystify many who pick up this book. After all, why should a general practitioner (GP) either need or want to own a pharmacy when there may well be one just down the street? What advantages can there possibly be to anyone by the arrangement? And anyway, don't the Regulations prevent it?

All these questions will be answered, but just take a look around you and you may well come across more than one practice that has an in-house pharmacy run by a pharmacist, but possibly owned by a doctors' company. It is becoming the vogue now, yet not so many years ago such services were extremely rare, if not totally non-existent. That is, until dispensing doctors began pre-empting a pharmacy attack in this way.

A brief history

Historically, the only practices that actually provided a full range of medicines to their patients were the dispensing practices. Many of the older, established, country practices of today were doing so long before there were chemists at all, let alone within practice premises. Included among them was my old practice in Welford, Northamptonshire. My original senior partner, the late Dr ACM Mann researched the practice back into the eighteenth century when our predecessors trotted around the neighbourhood on horseback with saddlebags stuffed with remedies.

The Pharmaceutical Society (PS) itself was not founded until the late nineteenth century and for very many years doctors and pharmacists coexisted peacefully, prescribing and dispensing relatively ineffective and inexpensive medicines. Pharmacy continued to show no real interest in the rural dispensing practices until drugs became much more effective in the 1920s. More effective drugs meant more expensive drugs and because chemists were paid on a 'cost-plus' basis, their profitability was increased. No longer were the rural areas so unattractive

In 1911, Lloyd-George instituted the 'one mile rule', following which patients living more than a mile from a chemist were allowed to choose whether to use the chemist or the dispensing practice. Over the years pharmacy has made many attempts to encroach upon, if not take over, the areas of dispensing practices and much acrimony developed between the two professions.

Another reason for the heightened interest of pharmacy in rural dispensing areas was caused by the appearance of the supermarket, which took away a great deal of the chemist's retail trade. Incidentally, the supermarkets are the direct cause of even greater concern for the chemists today and, for that matter, the appearance of this book, but more of that later. Back to the potted history of the provision of medicines to NHS patients.

The mid-1960s almost saw the complete destruction of the dispensing doctor and the invaluable service provided to rural patients. Government, pharmacists and the doctors' union – the General Medical Services Committee (GMSC) – seemed united in forcing through a destructive regulation. The 1966 Joint Working Party report would have allowed only patients with 'serious difficulty' in obtaining their medicines from a chemist, to get them from their doctor.

Enter Dr Gordon Scott of Milton-under-Wychwood who, on a cold foggy Sunday in November 1966, called an urgent ad hoc meeting of dispensing doctors to protest. Attendance from around the UK was 164. *The Times* ran a story on the meeting[1] and the Women's Institute joined the campaign at their annual conference that year. All parties retreated and doctor dispensing was saved, but the squabbles continued.

In 1984, The Clothier Regulations[2] – named after the chairman of the government enquiry team, Sir Cecil Clothier – were implemented. These regulations attempted to rigidly set out once and for all a procedure to determine which profession dispensed where.

Unfortunately, it was far from the cure that was intended. What it did do was to cause individual pharmacists and medical practices to examine the Regulations closely and to attempt to 'push the envelope' in their own favour. Dispensing applications by one side or the other seemed to proliferate and most went on to appeal. Nevertheless, on the whole there was an uneasy truce as the majority of both parties knew approximately where they stood.

The NHS maxim of 'The doctor shall prescribe and the chemist shall dispense each to their own special area of expertise' was always effectively quoted against applicant doctors wishing to dispense. No question then of 'shattering' professional boundaries. In the terms of the Regulations doctors did not provide 'pharmaceutical services', which is rather odd as the service they did provide – the provision of all drugs and appliances to their patients – is and was identical to that of the High Street chemist.

On the one side was the original Dispensing Doctors' Association (DDA), founded by the author in 1984 as a consequence of Clothier and other factors affecting dispensing practices, and on the other, a number of pharmacy organisations headed by the very large and professional National Pharmaceutical Association (NPA). Each fiercely defended its professional territory.

Before the DDA existed, dispensing doctors were largely without any protection because the General Medical Services Committee (GMSC) – now the General Practitioners Committee (GPC) – of the British Medical Association (BMA) amazingly let it be known that they were not there to defend any particular GP interest group – certainly not dispensing doctors. Maybe the memories of 1966 still rankled in Tavistock Square.

Suddenly, in the mid-1990s, a bombshell was dropped on the whole situation. An applicant pharmacist was told by the Appeal Authority that he was wasting his time, because he need not use the Clothier Regulations at all. Did he not know that there had been a misdrafting of the Act, which had been missed by the advisers of both professions?

As he already had a pharmacy within the health authority area, all that the chemist needed to do was to ask the authority for permission to set up a new shop, wherever he wished, within their area. He could ignore Clothier completely. The application would simply be considered under the 'necessary or desirable' clause of the Control of Entry Regulations for pharmacies.[3]

Remember that under the terms of the Regulations, dispensing practices do not provide pharmaceutical services. Therefore, if the authority thought a pharmacy was 'necessary or desirable to provide proper pharmaceutical services' it would be automatically granted permission.

As the chemist would not be applying if a colleague was already dispensing in that area, it followed that it was both necessary and desirable that the application should be granted.

This was the now infamous 'loophole' in Clothier and very many pharmacists have taken advantage of it over the last decade, at the same time creating even greater acrimony between the professions as scores of medical dispensing practices lost their dispensing rights – and the income that went with them – without any opportunity for a defence. And, of course, scores of pharmacy businesses were able to take over the dispensing businesses of another profession with the approval of the authorities and without having to pay a single penny in compensation. Small wonder that battle lines were drawn.

Despite extensive lobbying and pressure by the old DDA, successive governments refused to 'do the decent thing' and close the loophole to restore professional harmony. Relations worsened as legal actions taken by practices and the GMSC also largely failed. Even more dangerously for dispensing practices, in 1997, a schism was caused within the DDA, between those who wished to continue to press for closure of the loophole and those who wished to appease pharmacy by giving up even more rights in exchange for closure.

After a bitter legal wrangle the DDA appeasers won, despite Annual Conference resolutions two or three months previously, supporting the position of the others. The DDA was wound up and replaced by the DDA Ltd.

In 1997, the newly formed DDA Ltd decided that the way forward was to give pharmacy even more rights, if they agreed to join with the medical profession in asking government for a correction to the loophole. They proposed to unilaterally allow the future ring-fencing of dispensing by doctors by agreeing to the prohibition of further applications by potential dispensing practices in exchange for a slightly less effective protection for their dispensing colleagues. The chemists bit their hands off in their eagerness.

The GPC, the DDA Ltd and the pharmacists agreed to the changes and the necessary legislation was drafted some years ago. It is still being considered after a total of six years. And there the matter rests for the moment.

However, the whole matter of dispensing by doctors may well come under question during the government's current NHS reforms. For that very reason dispensing doctors should start seriously thinking about the viability of their practices, should this nightmare scenario come about.

This book is intended to indicate a way forward. It may be something of a volte-face for the original founder-chairman of the DDA, but medically owned pharmacies will keep dispensing where it belongs, in the surgery or health centre under the influence of those who know their patients best – the GPs.

The government, paradoxically, may be providing a lot of help for this future to be gained.

Recent changes – OFT and LIFT

One of the ways some dispensing doctors chose to protect their dispensing income from pharmacy applications was to do exactly what this book is about – to set up their own pharmacy by pre-empting such pharmacy applications. After all, who should know best about the viability of such a business but the dispensing practice? And who should know best whether an application would be imminently made by a pharmacist? Ask around your semi-rural colleagues and you may well come across an ex- or part-dispensing practice whose partners happily, and essentially, supplement their income from their own pharmacy.

They will be a source of great advice and help to any practice following in their footsteps. What they can do, you can do, and it has all been made much easier by recent government policies.

The NHS Plan[4] set out plans for radical changes throughout the NHS. This was clearly shown in Chapter 9, paragraph 9.5: 'The new approach will shatter the old demarcations which have held back staff and slowed down care'.

As this author should know, what stronger demarcations are there in the NHS than those between general practices and pharmacies, especially on the dispensing side. A blurring of the edges, loosening the dispensing regulations in favour of doctor dispensing would be welcomed by patients and doctors. There has been no such movement so far.

Elsewhere *The NHS Plan* (Executive Summary, page 11) says: 'Extra investment (will fund) ... 500 new one-stop primary care centres' and Chapter 8, paragraph 8.2: 'Up to 3000 family doctor premises including 500 new primary care centres will benefit from a £1 billion investment programme by 2004'.

The opportunity will be there for all the 3000 family doctor premises to be upgraded to provide facilities for other professions, perhaps to include a pharmacy.

As part of the 'shattering', Chapter 9, para. 9.8 of the Plan says:

> Pharmacists will be able to take on a new role as they shift away from being paid mainly for the dispensing of individual prescriptions towards rewarding overall service. Proposals will be invited for Personal Medical Services-type schemes that pilot alternative contracts for community pharmacy services. They will cover areas such as medicines management and repeat prescribing.

Pharmacists eagerly welcomed this and their movement into the actual prescribing of medicines, which was previously restricted to prescription only by doctors. Doctors, too, began to notice that the old NHS maxim about prescribing and dispensing, mentioned earlier, was being abandoned – at least for pharmacy.

Despite this small gap in the door, inexplicably neither the GPC nor the DDA Ltd has shown any interest in putting their shoulders to it to open it further. Quite the contrary, they have both been preoccupied with limiting doctor dispensing.

All seemed to be going well for pharmacy until along came a bombshell for them this time.

The large supermarket chains had been showing a keen interest in establishing their own in-house pharmacies for several years, but they were becoming frustrated and irritated by the restrictions imposed by the NHS 'control of entry regulations for pharmacy contracts'.

These include the Clothier Regulations and pharmacy Control of Entry Regulations as briefly mentioned above. What it boiled down to was – Is there already a pharmacy nearby and is there a need for another? Far too often the answers did not please the supermarket owners. Unless the supermarket was out of town on a greenfield site, there was almost certainly a high-street chemist within the statutory mile. Unfortunately for the supermarkets the tide had turned and greenfield site applications were no longer being granted for supermarket use. The result was that their applications for in-house pharmacies in their new urban supermarkets were being refused. Something had to be done.

Supermarket chains have big muscles and they used these to prevail upon the Office of Fair Trading[5] (OFT) to enquire into the control of entry regulations and the part these played in restricting fair trading in the pharmacy field.

The OFT examination was thorough and involved an investigation into the total provision of medicines throughout the community. As the current Regulations were designed specifically to restrict trade, the OFT had little choice but to suggest the total abandonment of the Regulations and thus allow a free-for-all. High-street chemists were to compete against high-street chemists *and* against the supermarkets. Any pharmacist – multiple or single – would be able to open a shop at will, anywhere – even, by the way, in rural areas. Deregulation would be, after all, deregulation. There was nothing for the doctors to cheer about.

The Fifth Report of the Session 2002–03 of the Commons Health Committee[6] in June 2003 also came down heavily upon dispensing by doctors by turning the clock back almost half a century to the 1966 Joint Working Party report, which had attempted to limit doctor dispensing to patients with exceptional difficulties. The Health Committee said:

> We recommend that the dispensing doctors' scheme is retained only where a pharmacy is unviable, even with the support of the Essential Small Pharmacy Scheme. Dispensing doctors should not be seen as a solution to problems arising from potential deregulation of entry into the market.

There was even less for doctors to cheer about, because unfortunately, the new DDA Ltd had failed to offer evidence to the Committee in defence of dispensing practice.

Pharmacy, it is safe to say, was very unhappy with this report, claiming that many high-street chemists would be forced out of business and NHS services would suffer. There is a flaw in this argument, but that will be left to the reader to find.

However, Mr D'Arcy[6] of the National Pharmaceutical Association (NPA), a witness to the Commons Health Committee in June 2003, over-egging matters as ever, insisted that the NPA thought between 800 and 900 pharmacies may be at risk if the Report was implemented as it stood.

Will this be 800–900 more opportunities for doctors' pharmacies to replace the high-street chemists?

After some months of consideration following the publication of the OFT report in January 2003, in July the Secretary of Trade for Industry, Patricia Hewitt, returned to pharmacy with her own new proposals,[7] which attempted to pacify both pharmacy and supermarket:

> ... pharmacies wishing to locate in shopping developments over
> 15 000 square metres in size will be exempt from the control of entry
> requirements.

> Similar arrangements and conditions will apply to pharmacies that
> intend to open for more than 100 hours a week, and to those that are
> part of a consortium to establish one of the new one-stop primary
> care centres proposed by my Rt. Hon. Friend the Secretary of State
> for Health.

So it appears that high-street pharmacies would continue to be regulated as before, but not pharmacies opening in developments of greater than 15 000 square metres, premises that remain open for 100 hours a week and, of interest to the readers of this book, those in one-stop healthcare premises.

The word 'new' is inserted before one-stop primary care centres, but that need not mean brand new. It could be interpreted as a health centre that has recently become a one-stop.

Lest some readers believe the author is too optimistic about the opportunities for medical practices, the following comment was written in *Pharmacy Magazine* by Mr David Reissner[8] of Charles Russell, a London firm of pharmacy-oriented solicitors, when discussing the government's amendments:

> What is a health centre? The government's proposals may accelerate
> the ownership of pharmacies by GPs − an undesirable development.

To answer Mr Reissner's question, according to *The NHS Plan* (Chapter 4, paragraph 4.12):

> New one-stop primary care centres will include GPs, dentists, opticians,
> health visitors, pharmacists and social workers.

So, remember what *The NHS Plan* said: '500 new one-stop primary care centres' and a promise to 'modernise 3000 GP premises'.

In itself that should create 3500 opportunities for alert and astute medical practices to get in first with their company application after having drawn up plans to allow for the inclusion of dentists, opticians and all the rest, *plus* a pharmacy.

In addition to those, there are many practices which, under the new GMS2 contract, are seeking to improve services to patients by including as many services under their own roof as possible. How silly it would be not to include a pharmacy and how exceedingly witless not to own that pharmacy themselves.

This book only refers to pharmacies, but many practices may well have the space to rent out to a visiting optician and dentist, thus creating the one-stop centre defined above and adding strength to the application for a pharmacy. It is fairly certain that the majority of practices already host health visitors.

Later chapters of this book may well persuade practices of the profitability of adding on extensions for these other services, assuming they have the space. The pharmacy would be an independently owned business whose shareholders would be the partners and the other professions would rent space from the GP.

Could it be that the need to chase tiresome GMS2 'brownie points' to maintain an income would be reduced? Few GPs would be sorry for that. Get planning!

It has to be said that the regulations are not yet in force, but close watching of the pharmacy scene has shown that government is indicating no intention to further modify its own modifications, despite pharmacy pressure.

Quite the contrary, in fact – Mrs Hewitt finished her response to the OFT report by saying: 'We will review progress in mid-2006, involving the OFT in this review, and publish our findings'.[7]

In March 2004, Health Minister Rosie Winterton seemed to reinforce this when she warned guests at a Pharmaceutical Society Negotiating Committee dinner that: '... we may disagree on just where we need to draw the lines'.

Emphasising their commitment to the changes, the government launched the new *NHS Improvement Plan*[9] for the NHS in England in July 2004 and promised that from the end of the year it would be easier to establish new pharmacies intending to open more than 100 hours a week, to operate wholly via mail order or the internet, or in one-stop primary care centres. But the fourth proposal outlined in the 'balanced package of measures' document – to allow new pharmacies to open in large shopping developments over 15 000 square metres floor space – was not mentioned.

The motto, therefore, is 'To the swiftest come the prizes', so be prepared.

As for dispensing practices – well, 10-metre high red neon lights are flashing furiously in your direction. You are potentially in great danger. Get your calculators out and if there is a glimmer of a possibility of your own pharmacy being a viability, get on with it. If you don't, then it's beginning to look as though sooner or later somebody will chop your head off. If you don't help yourself, there is nobody out there to help you.

As if that were not enough of an incentive for doctors to become interested in owning their own pharmacies, there is yet another player on the block. The NHS Local Improvement and Finance Trust (LIFT) – not totally unrelated to *The NHS Plan* – may well be almost as helpful as the OFT Report in the control of entry.

More practices may be able to relocate into an improved one-stop health centre with its own pharmacy, and pharmacists are already being warned that if they do not act together quickly the lease for that pharmacy may go to the highest bidder.

Could that be the medical practice? Pharmacist Steve Bremner, writing in the October 2003 *Pharmacy Magazine*[10], said:

> NHS LIFT is one of several models for funding improvements in the primary care estate that were announced in *The NHS Plan*. The government plans to invest £1 billion by 2004 and build 750 one-stop health centres by 2008. There are currently 42 designated LIFT areas, each containing between two and seven sites and 10 of these are already at the preferred bidder stage. They are mainly in areas of deprivation and cover 40% of PCTs.

> In LIFT areas a project team sets up a LIFT company (Liftco) which is 60% owned by a private sector partner that is appointed to work with the local health economy for 20 years. The Liftco then has exclusive

rights to tender for any new health and social care schemes within the area.

There are other regeneration initiatives that can be used to fund primary care estate, including the Neighbourhood Renewal Fund and New Deals for Communities. Development plans can be initiated by a variety of sources and utilise a range of funding but the PCT will co-ordinate operations and is a vital source of information.

All PCTs are being encouraged to develop a Strategic Service Development Plan (SSDP) which outlines a vision for primary care in their area for the next five to ten years and includes details of planned premises. PCTs can either work with local contractors to ensure that their SSDP includes provision for a stable pharmacy network that meets patient needs, or they can see pharmacy purely as a source of income through premises rental. The PCT's plans will depend largely on relationships with local contractors, representations made to them and the importance it places on developing pharmacy services.

All this is very revealing and very helpful to medical practices wishing to set up their own pharmacy company because nothing that Mr Bremner says can possibly be taken to exclude any pharmacy company, whoever owns it. The opening is there for doctors.

It has been said that government is opposed to companies of doctors owning pharmacies, but were they to attempt to restrict trade in this way it is almost certain that they would run foul of European Union (EU) legislation.

If deregulation means what it says, then, so far as one-stop primary care centres are concerned, under the modified OFT rules, the practice should only need to notify the primary care organisation (PCO) of what it is intending to do to become such a one-stop centre.

The vast majority of the practices mentioned above will be other than dispensing practices. However, dispensing practices in the present political climate, where, as we have seen, they have few friends, would be well advised to look out to their future security in a similar way.

Remember what the Commons Health Committee said:[6] 'We recommend that the dispensing doctors scheme is retained only where a pharmacy is unviable, even with the support of the ESP Scheme'.

Dispensing practices must hope that the GPC of the BMA and the DDA Ltd show more resolution in their defence than in the recent past.

At present there are 1565 dispensing practices, and more than 5000 dispensing doctors in the UK, 1242 of those practices being in England. Every one of those doctors and practices should now be sitting up and taking a very careful look around them. Are they ripe for the kill?

The 'loophole' has already been discussed and remains a massive danger to many practices as, indeed, do the present Clothier arrangements. These practices should keep an eye on their population size and density and their dispensing income. If both are increasing, then an application to pre-empt a pharmacy, either through Clothier, as described later in this book, or through the probable new OFT Regulations, may be advisable.

There are those who suggest that the pharmacy lobby is so powerful that the government will yield to the pressure and remove the one-stop primary care centres from the deregulation list.

The answer to this is that these centres are the flagship of primary care improvement and are mentioned many times in *The NHS Plan* and the government is unlikely to wish to see them scuppered.

Even if they do give way to pharmacy there will still be very many practices which own premises that can be readily adapted or extended. These partnerships will be the sole determinants as to who opens a pharmacy in those premises. The way to go about it is set out elsewhere in this book.

Why bother?

OK, so it looks very much as though it could be possible for any doctor-owned company to open a pharmacy without troubling the control of entry regulations but, some will ask, why bother? I have already told dispensing doctors why they should bother, but what about the rest of you?

The answer to that one could fill a book of its own, but an obvious answer is that a practice with its own pharmacy provides a full medical service to its patients. It will do this without the risk of the loss of confidentiality, which could occur if confidential medical histories were allowed to pass from surgeries to any number of high-street chemists, as is the intention under the presently discussed NHS plans.

Additionally, the patient may well buy their over-the-counter (OTC) medicines at the pharmacy, thus ensuring that the doctor has a full record of all medications taken by the patient. This must be a safety factor.

And, to be honest, there is the question of the increased income. If there has to be a pharmacy why let someone else profit from it being on your premises?

Alternatives

Some practices with space may wish to avoid all the possible hassle of running a pharmacy themselves. For them there are a number of alternatives and all of them profitable.

Assuming that there is space within the practice premises then the practice could advertise its availability for use as a pharmacy. There will be no need to place an advertisement in the local paper, but simply to write to a number of large pharmacy chains and it will not be long before you have a response – if not a stampede in your direction.

The addresses of all potentially interested companies are to be found in the *Chemist & Druggist Directory*,[11] but here are a few of the larger, national ones:

- AAH Retail Pharmacy Ltd (353 outlets), Osborn Way, Hook, Hampshire, RG27 9JA
- Boots the Chemists Ltd (1231 outlets), 1 Thane Road West, Nottingham, NG2 3AA
- Lloyds Chemists (899 outlets), Manor House, Manor Road, Mancetter, Atherstone, Warwickshire, CV9 1QY
- Moss E, Ltd (481 outlets), Fern Grove, Feltham, Middlesex, TW14 9BD

- National Co-operative Chemists Ltd (260 outlets), Brook House, Oldham Road, Middleton, Manchester, M24 1HF
- Unichem PLC (32 outlets), Unichem House, Cox Lane, Chessington, KT9 1SN.

In addition to these there are several companies which have a large number of shops in limited parts of the UK, such as:

- Northern Ireland
  - Bairds Chemists, (23 outlets), 159–161 Donegal Pass, Belfast, BT7 1DT
- Wales
  - Rowland & Co. (Retail) Ltd (68 outlets in Wales only), Dolydd Road, Wrexham, LL13 7TF
  - Howard & Palmer Ltd (29 outlets), Castell Close, Swansea Enterprise Park, Llansamlet, Swansea, SA7 9FH
- Kent
  - Paydens Ltd (30 outlets), Park Wood, Sutton Road, Maidstone, Kent ME15 9NN
- Lancashire and Cheshire
  - Gorgemead Ltd (44 outlets), Unit L, Kershaw Business Centre, Bolton, Lancashire, BL3 5BF
  - United Norwest Healthcare (65 outlets), Leader House, Greenfield Road, Greenfield Business Park, Congleton, Cheshire, CW12 4TR
- Scotland
  - Red Band Chemical Co Ltd (18 outlets), T/A Lindsay & Gilmour Chemist, 19 Smiths Place, Edinburgh, EH6 8NU.

The above lists are very far from being exhaustive. Once again, the annual *Chemist & Druggist Directory* has a complete list of all multiples with more than five shops in their chain. By definition there is bound to be such a chain close to every surgery. Buy, beg, borrow or steal a copy of the *Directory* and get those letters off.

Before writing to offer your premises, be sure of your facts and it would be helpful if the local authority (LA) was approached to check on planning permission for the change of use to a retail outlet of that part of your surgery.

Chapter 2 – Will the pharmacy be viable? – should help you to calculate a reasonable estimate of the profit to be expected from the pharmacy.

In addition, review your prescribing figures for the past few years and work on that to provide a suitable figure. Then remember to include a factor for retail sales, as covered in Chapter 2.

Bearing all this in mind, be very careful about the contract you draw up with the chemist. As you will see, there is a great deal of profit to be made. As a start, just look at your Prescribing Analysis and CosT data (PACT) and other prescribing figures provided by the PCT. Why do you think so much pressure is being exerted upon you about your prescribing? Come to that, when did you last see a poor urban chemist?

The chains will bring some big guns to bear on you, but you are the one with the figures. You know what renting the premises is worth and it will be worth a great deal. If you are not sure, then ask your accountant for help.

It is at this stage that you should approach your solicitor for advice about contracts.

Get into a Dutch auction and consider either a straight rental or rental plus a profit share. The latter is likely to be more advantageous. When renting out your premises remember to include a clause covering regular and frequent reviews. If this is the way you choose to go, then you have a golden opportunity. Do not squander that opportunity.

Alternatively, you may have been friendly with the independent chemist down the road for the past 20 years, so give him a chance, too. But even if you play golf with him, remember that he is a business man – and so are you. Business rules apply. If he's worth his salt, he will expect nothing less.

Of course, if the potential OFT deregulation changes come into effect then your local high-street pharmacist, be he an owner or manager, may be interested to understand that a pharmacy established in the primary care premises is likely to attract pretty well all the dispensing of the practice. That should increase the bargaining power of the practice, but should not lead to any unemployment of pharmacists. There is a shortage of pharmacists and any made redundant in the high street could well find employment in the primary care health centre.

What about selling OTCs?

Chapter 12 will deal with this subject in full.

Selling OTCs is a slight divergence from the main topic of the book, but there may be some doctors who don't want to go the whole way and open a pharmacy. They could open a dispensary. It is, of course, much simpler to restrict sales to OTCs because there are no regulations involved, other than retail, so long as *pharmacy only* and *prescription only* medicines are avoided.

Any practice can sell OTCs if they set up a separate dispensary company to do so. Otherwise, they cannot sell to their own NHS patients. Advice on how to set up a company is given in Chapter 5. The general rules are the same, whether it is a pharmacy company or a dispensary.

Dispensing practices are an exception to this rule. When Kenneth Clarke brought in the NHS prescription 'black list' (Section XVIII of *The Drug Tariff*)[12] in 1984 he was made to realise by the DDA that rural patients would be put at a disadvantage by not being able to obtain many of these commonly used medicines. The result was a change to the NHS Medical and Pharmaceutical Regulations to allow, for the first time, an NHS GP to sell medicines to their patients.

> A doctor may prescribe such (Schedule 3A) items privately though he may not charge for doing so and can sell such items only if he is a doctor entitled under the 1974 Regulations to dispense to a patient and then only to that patient in respect of a course of treatment.

There is a later requirement to 'keep a record in the patient's notes'. This is now interpreted as implying that there must be no charge for a private prescription form, all OTCs sold must be listed in *The Drug Tariff* and that electronic records may be kept.

A significant number of dispensing practices have used this freedom to sell these medicines – and other retail goods – as one of their strategies to protect their dispensing service from the ingression of a pharmacy. Their patients and the village shopkeepers, being aware of the danger to their own trade, have sometimes set up a joint venture.

It is essential that only experienced dispensers should sell the medicines in these dispensaries and that they should always advise the patient to see the doctor if the symptoms persist or if there is any doubt. The same should apply in community pharmacy.

In dispensing practices any medicine may be sold under the doctor's supervision, whether it is pharmacy only, prescription only or on the general sales list (GSL), just so long as it is blacklisted. There are upwards of 3000 preparations in Section XVIII and the list is growing almost daily.

Chapter 12 lists the many safeguards suggested to protect patients, staff and doctors:

- keep records
- ensure the computer is updated with the blacklist status of drugs
- review self-treatment protocols
- review 'repeats' if needed
- use the computer to cross-check for compatibility with prescribed drugs
- keep records.

The benefits of retail OTC medicines being available at the surgery or dispensary are very many and they apply to patients, the NHS, doctors and even to pharmacies.

If this idea is beginning to appeal, then it is worth flicking forward now to Chapter 12 where they are all set out.

Practices providing this service have many unique selling points (USPs), which encourage their patients to buy from them rather than from elsewhere, and it is worth listing them now. The practice:

- is in the right place at the right time
- has a captive clientele
- has the patient's drug and medical history available to cross-check
- can always assess the safety of the OTC with current prescribed drugs
- runs an efficient dispensary
- has qualified staff
- has a complete range of effective products recommended by the doctor
- has free in-house publicity through the practice leaflet
- is able to price competitively.

Most of the benefits listed above apply even more if the practice runs its own pharmacy from within the practice and much of the advice offered elsewhere in this book applies to the setting up of an independent dispensary. So, please read on.

Summary

Already, many practices are in a position to set up their own, in-house pharmacy, but recent NHS changes and potential changes will increase the opportunities immensely. General practices are in the best position to take advantage of all these because they know best whether such a venture would be viable.

Theoretically, the NHS is not interested in who owns the pharmacy, but they are very interested that it should be efficiently and safely run for the health and convenience of their patients. The pharmacist that the practice company employs can do this just as well as a high-street pharmacist. Indeed, they may be the same. It is possible that if a high-street chemist closes under the potential OFT Rules (although unlikely) the practice pharmacist may be literally the same person.

There is no doubt that patients will appreciate an in-house pharmacy. Doubters should just ask all those patients of dispensing practices what they think. They should especially ask the patients who, following a successful pharmacy application, can no longer get their medicines at the doctor's.

As for the doctors, they should be happier with the increased income and the reduced need to chase quality and other 'bean-counting' points in the new GMS2 contract.

So, there are the motives and the opportunities. All you have to do is to commit the deed. Chapter 3 onwards will, I hope, guide you through the process to a successful conclusion – be it under current regulations or new ones.

As for the alternatives – well, that is just what they are. Far better to go the whole hog yourself. Think of the satisfaction to be gained by your patients – and yourselves. Not to mention the inevitably improved safety of the close relationship between practice and pharmacy. And you will have the satisfaction of carrying out government policy, too.

References

1   *Dispensing Plan Opposed.* 25 September 1966, *The Times,* London.
2   *NHS (General Medical & Pharmaceutical Services) Amendment Regulations 1983, No. 313 (Clothier Regulations).* Stationery Office, London.
3   *The NHS (Pharmaceutical Services) Regulations 1992 (Control of Entry Regulations).* Stationery Office, London.
4   Department of Health (2000) *The NHS Plan.* Stationery Office, London.
5   Office of Fair Trading (2003) *The Control of Entry Regulations and Retail Pharmacy Services in the UK.* OFT, London.
6   Commons Health Committee (2003) *The Fifth Report of the Session 2002–03.* Stationery Office, London.
7   Hewitt P (July 2003) *Parliamentary Statement on Community Pharmacies.* Stationery Office, London.
8   Reissner D (2004) Talking point. *Pharmacy Magazine.* **January:** 6.
9   Department of Health (2004) *The NHS Improvement Plan.* Stationery Office, London.
10 Bremner S (2003) Ready for LIFT off? *Pharmacy Magazine.* **September:** 6.
11 *Chemist & Druggist Directory* (published annually by CMP Data & Information, Tonbridge).
12 Department of Health (updated regularly) *The Drug Tariff.* Stationery Office, London.

Chapter 2

Will the pharmacy be viable?

Before getting down to the nitty-gritty of putting in the application, a not unimportant question is to consider whether your new pharmacy will be viable. Surprisingly, not all pharmacies are. The exceptional ones may be in the small minority, but there is absolutely no point in establishing a pharmacy that is going to become a financial millstone for years to come, that is, unless yours is a dispensing practice threatened by a pharmacy application. In that case, better, perhaps, to make a small loss through your own pharmacy than suffer the total loss of your dispensing income.

It is a fact, as will be described later, that where the NHS through the PCT considers a pharmacy to be essential, it will subsidise it through the Essential Small Pharmacy Scheme (ESPS) to provide the pharmacist with a bare minimum income.

Mr D'Arcy of the NPA is quoted in the Commons Health Committee, Fifth Report, 2002–03, saying:[1]

> The Essential Small Pharmacy Scheme has been proposed as an alternative, but it is not a credible alternative or a way of solving the closure problem, because it is essentially a top-up payment, and it is not a particularly good one. It will keep the pharmacy afloat, but it does not turn it into a good pharmacy practice.

He continues:

> ... we have opined that there could be between 800 and 900 pharmacies at risk – if they were to be supported by the ESPS, it is untenable to suggest that the current arrangements, where the subsidy is taken from other pharmacy contractors' remuneration – that is not tenable as an alternative.

So, it might or might not be all very well for pharmacists, but many readers will see little point in a doctor-owned company having such a hand-to-mouth existence unless, of course, it is a threatened dispensing practice with all to lose.

It is probably far better to let the existing high-street chemist exist in peace. Alternatively, if the practice has surplus space then it could offer it to the pharmacist, as mentioned earlier, at a respectable rent. The choice will be yours.

Before calculating the back-of-an-envelope profitability of your pharmacy a decision must be made as to what services it will provide. Will it simply be a dispensing pharmacy or will it stock retail goods and, if so, to what extent? In addition to those two services, many pharmacies these days provide a number of diagnostic tests at a fee to the patient. Pregnancy tests, cholesterol tests and blood pressure monitoring are three that immediately come to mind. There are several others.

Having said that, it is just possible that as the pharmacy is so closely allied – logistically if not by name – to the surgery there may be some reluctance from patients to pay for tests which might otherwise be provided by the NHS.

Will the NHS dispensing be profitable?

The answer to that will almost certainly be an emphatic 'yes', unless the practice is in a very rural area where a pharmacy may need the help of the Essential Small Pharmacy Scheme.

The practice itself is in the best position to be able to calculate just how profitable a new pharmacy could be. After all, the doctors – and nurses, these days – are the ones who actually prescribe the drugs that generate the profit for the pharmacy. And do not forget the increasing prescribing activities of the pharmacist as well.

Another vital factor is that an in-house pharmacy will catch virtually all the prescriptions generated by the practice, because it will be so conveniently placed, even if there were a remaining high-street pharmacy. That also includes the sales of OTC medicines if the pharmacy decides to provide them.

Why else would community pharmacies be so anxious about the relaxing of the pharmacy contract entry regulations?

Before going into the finances in great detail, doctors should be aware that for generations potentially disadvantaged high-street pharmacies have levelled the accusation at dispensing practices that they 'prescribe to line their own pockets'. There is no reason to believe that this accusation will change when a doctors' consortium owns the pharmacy.

Be aware of this and keep a close eye, as ever, on the practice prescribing figures. Yes, I know, the PCT already does it for you and it is always very ready to raise an especially heavy hand in the direction of the practice if the budget falls outside the PCT averages. This has been the justified retort from every dispensing doctor to his pharmacy detractors.

Pharmacy income
NHS income

It is important to separate out the income from fees and from stock prescribed items. The regular form FP 34 will help this because all fees are displayed on it for analysis. *The Drug Tariff*[2] carries all the fees and it is itemised below.

Also on the FP 34 are the drug costs. Allowance should be made for the Prescription Pricing Authority (PPA), PPA/PCO discount clawback and other expenses, to leave reasonably accurate figures for the drugs dispensed.

Many of the sources of pharmacy income from the NHS are set out in *The Drug Tariff* but, of course, not everyone has a copy to hand and, in any case, it is a very wearisome book to get into. Those who may not yet have closely examined a copy should be warned that it is a softback A5 book, which appears to be set in

Arial 6pt or smaller. The whole thing simply screams out, 'Don't bother to read me, I'm boring and useless'.

It is not useless and the dispensing doctor or pharmacist who takes it at its word and bins it is a very foolish professional indeed. *The Drug Tariff* is one of the most useful and essential works provided by the NHS. New editions containing details of payments, permitted appliances and preparations, together with other information changed since the previous edition, are published and distributed every month.

Ignore what *The Drug Tariff* says at your financial peril. Even if you need matchsticks to prop your eyelids open, read it carefully. Especially concentrate on the first few pages where the most recent changes are to be found.

Sources of income

1 *Drug Tariff* payments/fees
   - Preface: amendments
   - Part II: calculation of payments
   - Part IIIA/B: professional fees – pharmacy and appliance contractors
   - Part IV: containers
   - Part V: deduction scale
   - Part VIA: additional professional services
   - Part VIC: repeat dispensing fees
   - Part VIII: basic prices of drugs
   - Part IX: appliances
   - Part X: domiciliary oxygen
   - Part XI: additional pharmacist access services
   - Part XII: the Essential Small Pharmacies Scheme
   - Part XIII: payment in respect of pre-registration trainees
   - Part XIVA: advice to care homes
   - Part XIVB: patient medication records
   - Part XIVC: fraudulent prescription forms
   - Part XVIIIA: substances not to be prescribed on the NHS.
2 the profit between purchase and repayment prices
3 OTC sales
4 private and NHS-paid diagnostic services
5 retail sales
6 miscellaneous sources of income.

Each of these will be described in some detail below.

The Drug Tariff
Preface: amendments
Having read the book thoroughly once to get it into your system, this section is probably, serially, the most important because it sets out the monthly changes. It begins by providing the symbols that appear throughout the text to indicate price rises, reductions and other changes, such as additional products or changes to the acceptable specifications.

Readers must constantly bear in mind that if a product is not listed in the Tariff it is not acceptable to the NHS and payment will not be made for it. Even worse than that, in 1984, Health Secretary Kenneth Clarke made it a punishable offence for a contractor to attempt to provide 'disallowed' items on an NHS prescription form. However, to our knowledge no one has ever suffered whatever penalty there may be for doing that. It is believed that offenders were to have been referred to what was then called a 'Service Committee', for which read 'disciplinary' committee.

The pharmacist must be constantly aware of this in order to refer a prescription back to the prescribing doctor if necessary. His income depends on it.

Part II: calculation of payments

A word of caution. The current payment system is described below but the new pharmacy contract may well drastically change this. However, it is extremely unlikely that any pharmacist will be less well paid under any new system.

Dispensing doctors may not know that the payment scheme for pharmacists differs from their own. There are moves afoot to align the dispensing doctor scheme with pharmacy.

Each prescription item is paid for in the following way:

1   The price of the drug (A)

Less

2   An amount based on the total price of drugs submitted, calculated from Part V, the Deduction Scale (q.v.) (B)

And

3   the appropriate professional fee (Part IIIA, q.v.) (C)

And

4   the container allowance (Part IV, q.v.) (D)

So, the reimbursed price per item $= (A - B) + C + D$

Part II goes on to describe other payments and the endorsement (of prescriptions) requirements.

Among the other payments are:

- *broken bulk* – This applies to drugs, appliances and chemical reagents where the quantity ordered on the prescription is less than the quantity that must be purchased and where the remainder may not be easily disposed of without loss. It does not apply across the board to every prescription item.
- *out-of-pocket expenses* – An additional fee will be paid where the pharmacist has incurred exceptional expenses in obtaining a preparation. For instance, it may have been necessary to visit a hospital pharmacy to complete a prescription that a doctor has written for an unusual preparation, according to a hospital consultant's directions.
- *the zero discount list* – The NHS assumes that all dispensing doctors and pharmacists purchase the drugs they supply to the NHS at a discount and, through their respective deduction ('clawback') scales a large portion of this discount is paid to the NHS.

  However, pharmacists and dispensing doctors are unable to obtain a discount when purchasing a considerable number of products. *The Drug Tariff* currently

lists around 250 such items and the NHS does not in
pharmacy discount deduction scale. Instead, it places them
Discount (ZD) list. No discount clawback is deducted fr
from this list if the prescription is endorsed 'ZD'.

For some very odd, unaccountable reason that infuriate
there is no such ZD scheme for them and discount that th
deducted from them. Maybe that will be tidied up if the dispensing
payment system ever becomes similar to the pharmacists' scheme. But that is by
the way!

The money is deducted at source by the PPA.

Part IIIA/B: professional fees

Prescription fee – Currently (March 2004) all prescriptions attract a fee of 94.60p.
A 'prescription' means each item on every FP 10. 'Now, doctor, how many items
did you write last month?' It is simple to find that out and quite easy to multiply
that by 94.6p. It will amount to a tidy sum.

Additional fees – There are several classes of 'extemporaneously dispensed' prescriptions, which attract an additional fee each. 'Extemporaneously dispensed'
means that the preparation is actually made up in the dispensary, but these are few
and far between nowadays, because few doctors write detailed prescriptions as
most items are manufactured. The current fee varies between 85p and £7.67p
according to the class of item.

'Appliances and dressings' are quite commonly prescribed and attract an additional
fee of between 69p and £1.97p (for a truss).

'Call out' fees are paid when the pharmacist dispenses out of hours. This varies
between £7.13 and £21.18 according to the circumstances and whether the doctor
endorses the script 'urgent'.

Part IV: containers

Pharmacists and dispensing doctors must supply medicines in a 'suitable container' of the description demanded in *The Drug Tariff*. Payment for the container
is 3.24p, whether the item is prepacked by the manufacturer or individually
dispensed in a container provided by the pharmacist.

Part V: deduction scale

Pharmacists and dispensing doctors are both assumed to be astute business people
who manage to purchase drugs at a discount from the manufacturer directly, from
their wholesaler, or both. The NHS believes that this is unjust and demands its
share. Each profession has its own discount deduction scale.

The scale varies according to the value of the total number of items submitted
to the PPA each month. The greater the number submitted, the greater the percentage 'clawback' on the total number of items, except ZD items, in the case of
pharmacists. There are multiple steps in the scale, which is regularly reviewed by
detailed 'Discount enquiries'.

At a total value of the prescriptions submitted to the PPA of up to £125/month
the deduction is currently at a rate of 5.93% and where that total value exceeds
£150 001/month, the rate maximises at 12.52%. For interest's sake, that works out
at a deduction of £18 780.13p for one month alone.

As dispensing doctors have found, it is an essential, tail-chasing exercise to maximise discounts. Chapter 10 covers the purchase of stock.

Part VIA: additional professional services

If the pharmacy has produced a practice leaflet, displayed a maximum of eight health promotion leaflets and keeps patient medication records, an additional fee will be paid according to the number of prescription items they dispense. The fee varies from £755 per month for between 1100 and 1600 items to a maximum of £1460 per month if more than 1600 items are dispensed per month.

Part VIC: repeat dispensing fee

More and more chemists are becoming 'repeat dispensing chemists' and this service attracts a start-up fee of £150 and a monthly payment of £100. A 'repeat dispensing chemist' endeavours, with the agreement of the prescribing doctor, to monitor patients whose drugs are on regular repeat prescriptions.

Part VIII: basic prices of drugs

This is not an additional fee but simply a list of prices determined by the Secretary of State, according to pack size. The list is in four categories: readily available drugs; drugs with declining usage; drugs priced on the basis of a particular brand or manufacturer; and extemporaneously prepared items.

It is important that the pharmacist is aware of this section as many scripts have to be endorsed in particular ways to ensure correct and prompt payment by the PPA. The list covers 50 pages of the Tariff.

Part IX: appliances

This is a very important section, especially as the list of approved appliances seems to change monthly. Check the Preface! The section takes up 325 Tariff pages. Each and every item is detailed and costed, many with information regarding the approved supplier. If a doctor prescribes an item that has subsequently been removed from the list, that item will not be paid for by the PPA.

Part X: domiciliary oxygen

At an early stage in planning a decision must be taken on whether to supply domiciliary oxygen. It is a useful and profitable service but, as would be expected, special precautions must be made for the storage of cylinders and equipment. Approval must be sought from the PCT before the service can be provided. Careful thought should be given before applying. The application will need the support of the local pharmaceutical committee, which closely monitors the provision of oxygen services to the community.

Part XI: additional pharmacist access services

This fee replaces the original Rota Service and is decided between the pharmacist and the PCT.

Part XII: the Essential Small Pharmacies Scheme (ESPS)

This is only relevant to the smaller, rural pharmacies and it is unlikely, perhaps, that many of the pharmacies being discussed in this book will qualify for it. But, it is a fee and is described for completeness.

Only pharmacies that dispense fewer than 24 360 prescriptions per year will qualify for the payment. In addition they must be more than one kilometre from the next nearest pharmacy. It is also essential that they have a practice leaflet and display eight health promotion posters. There are several other conditions described in *The Drug Tariff*. The amount paid is a maximum of £2990 per month, calculated according to an NHS formula.

Part XIII: payment in respect of pre-registration trainees

Pharmacists who provide appropriate training for pharmacy graduates before the graduates are accepted on to the Pharmaceutical Society's Register are paid at an annual rate of £4910 per student.

Part XIVA: advice to care homes

A fee is payable according to certain circumstances as detailed in *The Drug Tariff*. They broadly consist of advising the care home on:

• the proper and effective ordering of drugs and appliances for the residents
• the proper and effective administration of drugs and appliances to the residents
• the safe and appropriate storage of the drugs.

The chemist must keep a record of the services provided and make that record available to the authority on request.

Part XIVB: patient medication records

If the records of two categories of patients are kept by the pharmacist a fee will be provided. The categories are men and women over 60 years of age and others whom the pharmacist considers may have difficulty in understanding the nature and dosage of their drugs. There are other conditions. The set-up fee is £300 for new patient medication record systems.

Part XIVC: fraudulent prescription forms

Once again this is a fee that will be attracted by few of the described pharmacies in this book for the obvious reasons that the prescriptions will mostly be generated in the surgery and a bare minimum of prescriptions will be brought in from outside sources.

The vast majority of fraud is committed by patients attempting to obtain illicit medicines or to avoid the prescription charge, which is currently £6.30 per item. After a period of time the chemist and his staff will have entered the exempt or otherwise details on the computer system and may even know the patients personally.

The fee paid, under certain carefully set-out conditions, will be £70 per case.

Part XVIIIA: substances not to be prescribed on the NHS

This is otherwise known as the 'Black List' and was introduced by Health Secretary Kenneth Clarke MP in 1984. In those days there were relatively few items on it, but now the list covers 30 pages and includes around 3500 items.

The list is mentioned if only to remind readers that if an item from it is submitted to the PPA payment will be disallowed. This will mean a loss of both the cost of the medicine and the various dispensing fees.

As an aside, dispensing doctors should be aware that they may sell any item from this list to their dispensing patients – a point of interest that should tempt many to set up an OTC sales service (*see* Chapters 1 and 12).

More details of these Drug Tariff services will be found in Chapter 11.

The profit between purchase and repayment prices

This is where business sense and acumen comes in with a vengeance. Some have it and some do not, but it is of major, if not crucial importance. A factor that should spur everybody on is Part V of *The Drug Tariff*, the discount deduction scale. As previously mentioned, the NHS takes it for granted that the contracting pharmacy will be obtaining the greatest discount, or best deal, possible and it demands its share.

That share is over 12.5% on a total submission of £150 000. Other expenses to be deducted from that sum will be described later in this chapter and all of them reduce the profit margin.

There is a current series of Channel 4 television programmes where the subject of the programme buys a property for renovation in the hope of selling it on at a profit. A budget is drawn up, following an attempt to cost out the various stages and parts of the process. Advice is given throughout by an expert presenter. Almost universally the subjects allow outside and personal influences to exceed the budget and reduce the profit margin. This should not, but can easily happen to the unwary new owners of a pharmacy, or any other business – so beware.

Reimbursement prices

The first matter is to understand at what price the PPA will reimburse the dispenser.

Section VIII (q.v.) of *The Drug Tariff* contains several pages of basic prices of drugs. Other prices have been agreed by the NHS with the manufacturer under the Prescription Price Regulation Scheme and can be obtained from the PPA.

The Monthly Index of Medical Specialities (MIMS) gives the NHS price, which is the cost price excluding VAT. This is the price upon which the prescribers' PACT figures are based.

Purchase price of drugs and medicines

These are determined by the business skills of the purchasing manager, be that one of the partners or, one hopes, more usually, the pharmacist in charge.

As previously mentioned, discounts are there to be made in this very odd world where they are provided only so that the Department of Health can largely remove them from the pharmacy.

A wise pharmacist will be well aware of the monthly income of the pharmacy generated by drug reimbursements. He will also know how much discount, in percentage terms, is being deducted by the PPA or PCT and the discount he demands from his suppliers should exceed that comfortably.

This is not the place to advise readers how to obtain discounts or from where to obtain them. That will be dealt with later. Suffice to know that there is a great deal of help provided, not to mention a multitude of price lists from a multitude of suppliers.

Over-the-counter sales

Although by far the largest part of the pharmacy income will be generated by NHS services, including dispensing, over-the-counter (OTC) sales of medicines can be responsible for a reasonable profit level.

Unlike drug stores or dispensaries, which do not need a superintendent pharmacist and are limited in what they can sell, pharmacies may sell any medicine except prescription only medicines (POMs). It must be said that there are moves afoot, however unwise they may be, to allow chemists to sell even some current POMs. One has to assume that the powers that be compiled the POM list after careful thought and for good reason and, therefore, to wonder at the mindset behind these proposals.

To help sales along many manufacturers advertise extensively on television and, before doing so, give advance notice to the chemist when the advertisement will appear. This allows the pharmacy to stock up. Details of the various campaigns are given, from time to time, in *Chemist & Druggist* magazine, the retail magazine for pharmacy.

It is becoming essential for 'Pharmacy Only' sales to be made by specially trained staff. Members of the Association of Pharmacy Technicians (APT) (*see* Chapter 7) will have been trained to a high level as a condition of membership.

It is regrettable that the old habit of the shop assistant thrusting her hand in the air clutching a paper bag while nodding to the distant pharmacist for permission to sell, is still with us. No medically owned pharmacy should permit this. The prime objective should be patient safety.

Private and NHS-paid diagnostic services

For some years now pharmacists have been seeking to increase their range of activities from simply dispensing or selling medicines and other goods. Diagnostic services come readily to mind. The long list below is being added to by the day by entrepreneurial pharmacists.

If full advantage is to be taken of this opportunity it is essential that there be a separate and quiet area for the customer/patient to be interviewed and perhaps tested. Few people will be happy to bare their arms, or other parts of their anatomy, in a crowded shop. It should not be too difficult for a shop-fitter or designer to create such a space in the new pharmacy (*see* Chapter 8).

A number of tests amongst the list below may well be carried out for a fee paid either by the NHS or privately by the patient.

Some of the 'near patient' diagnostic tests and health monitoring services that may be provided either now or in the near future are:

- blood pressure
- cholesterol
- lipid profile
- diabetes: HbA1c, creatinine, glucose, ketones
- weight and height
- pregnancy
- therapeutic drug monitoring
- biochemical monitoring
- anticoagulant monitoring: INR warfarin
- asthma monitoring

- chronic obstructive pulmonary disease monitoring
- helicobacter pylori eradication
- body mass index (BMI).

It is predicted that it will not be long before the following are profitably added to that list:

- glycated haemoglobin
- microalbuminuria
- haemostasis
- urinary tract infections: leucocytes, protein, blood, nitrite
- streptococcus A
- glandular fever
- urea and electrolytes, bilirubin, urobilinogen, specific gravity
- faecal occult blood
- osteoporosis screening.

It is possible that a few pharmacists can add to this list, but the above are the more common services provided. Current fee levels may be suggested by the NPA, the trade organisation for pharmacists, of which every pharmacist should be a member.

To summarise, the new opportunities for diagnostic or near-patient services include:

- in-pharmacy diagnostic services
- retailing self-management products
- retailing disease management products
- medicine management services
- repeat prescribing and dispensing management.

And don't forget travel services – medicines, vaccines, equipment, all of them being opportunities for income enhancement.

As the pharmacy being described here will be within primary care premises where many tests can be provided by the NHS, maybe the income from this source will be rather limited.

Alert GPs will have noticed that among the above list are a number of tests that could well be described, for the sake of the new GP contract, as 'enhanced services' which, of course, attract an income for the doctors.

Under the terms of the new pharmacy contract, whose implementation has been delayed until October 2004 at least, the tests may be available for the pharmacy to bid for a PCO contract for their provision in competition with the GPs.

It may well be worth investigating which would be the most profitable contractor – your company pharmacy or the medical practice, that is, if the opportunity remains when the pharmacy is up and running.

Retail sales
Retail sales cover everything from pharmacy-only and GSL medicines to the non-medical, from hot water bottles, to cameras, films and, even in some cases, alcohol. The Royal Pharmaceutical Society of Great Britain prohibits the sale of tobacco in pharmacies.

However, that apart, it is down to the owners of the pharmacy what they sell, just so long as that does not conflict with pharmacy or medical ethics. That being so, then the income from this source may be small or large.

Most in-house pharmacies will, perhaps, have little room or scope for many items other than drugs. Herbal preparations may interest some, but they should be carefully selected as having some value as well as being safe.

Miscellaneous sources of income

There are a few of these but I do expect a shoal of letters from pharmacists eager to add to my meagre list of counselling, hypnotherapy (if trained) and certificate signing. Readers should not think of this as being a major source of profits.

Conclusion

There should be no problem at all for a pharmacy established within primary care premises to exist profitably on the income from NHS dispensing alone plus a few sales over the counter of the more common items. In fact, if the pharmacy is within an urban or semi-rural area, then it should be able to capture virtually all of the NHS dispensing generated by the surgeries.

That being so, there should be no need for the sale of retail products and near-patient testing could be reserved as an NHS service, other than in exceptional circumstances where NHS tests are unavailable. The choice is yours.

Pharmacy expenses

This section is not meant to be a closely detailed list of every expense incurred running a pharmacy. Instead, it is intended to cover the most obvious expenses involved in establishing the pharmacy and some of the running costs. A comparison may then be made with the estimate of the income generated.

For the sake of argument, and it will be correct in virtually all cases, it is being assumed that the primary care premises will either have to build an extension or modify the existing building. Before doing so it is good sense to consult the Pharmaceutical Society for advice on the minimum size of the premises after paying a discrete visit to existing pharmacies.

One-off expenses

- Planning including local authority, architects and solicitors' fees.
- Building.
- Modifying premises.
- Shop-fitting.
- Stocking with professional equipment.
- Initial stocking with all goods.

Ongoing expenses

- Staff salaries – pharmacist, including part-time and/or locum pharmacist.
- Dispensing assistant(s).

- Shop assistant(s).
- Subscriptions to professional bodies and insurance organisations.
- Rent and 'rates'.
- Heating, lighting, water.
- Discount deduction scale (*The Drug Tariff*).
- Restocking – prescription and OTC.

For the sake of argument it will be assumed that the practice has sufficient space already to convert to accommodate a pharmacy. Obviously, planning, building and other costs for those who have to start from scratch are infinitely variable and beyond the scope of this guide.

Once again, such one-off expenses as shopfitting and equipping the pharmacy are also variable. Some indication of the costs involved may be obtained by contacting a number of pharmacy shopfitters for an estimate.

The names below are picked at random from that inestimable annual publication – *The Chemist & Druggist Directory*[3] – where a much more complete list may be found. It should be emphasised that there is no personal recommendation for any firm mentioned.

- Barlow Shopfitting Ltd, South Yorkshire – 0114 255 6331
- Beanstalk, Northamptonshire – 01933 401555
- CIL International Ltd, London – 0171 272 0222
- Gemma Shopfitting Systems, Dorset – 01305 257888

The same publication lists virtually all the suppliers of equipment needed to run a pharmacy according to RPS regulations. A list of suggested equipment is to be found in Chapter 8.

Recurring expenses

Of these the most important are staff salaries and expenses. For most businesses they are the greatest overhead and it is worthwhile thinking of them as a separate item. If profitability is not as high as expected, then some tinkering about with staff costs may remedy the problem. There is usually some flexibility here. When tempted to tinker in this way always remember the employment laws and if you do not remember them, then look them up again. Your time will not be wasted.

The pharmacist

At the outset it must be understood that no pharmacy can operate unless there is a pharmacist actually on the premises all the time. That is the law and there is no getting around it. How long it will remain the law is debatable, because there are strong moves afoot to relax it so that pharmacists can leave the premises to undertake new roles in the community, such as visiting the elderly to supervise medication and visiting post-operative patients.

However, for the time being a pharmacist is essential 100% of the time, which brings into urgent consideration the matters of opening hours and how many hours the superintendent pharmacist will work.

The in-house pharmacy should be open at the very least to cover surgery hours, together with Saturdays and maybe even Sunday availability. Assuming the pharmacist has a working week of 37 hours, that must mean that more than one is required. The suggestion is one full-time plus a part-timer on a rota system. Then, do not forget holiday periods and sickness when locum pharmacists will be needed.

There are various figures suggested for the salary of a full-time pharmacist. About £30 000–£40 000 per annum appears to be mid-scale. Locum fees may be around £200+ per day.

The pharmacist will probably wish to be a member of the NPA and will have to be a member of the RPSGB. The company may wish to pay these subscriptions.

Dispensers

Although, rather surprisingly, there is as yet no legal requirement to employ trained dispensers, it is obviously good practice to do so. Their salary scale is based on the Whitley Council rates. Details of these are to be found in current editions of *Medeconomics*,[4] from nearby dispensing practices or from the Association of Pharmacy Technicians (APT), (q.v.). Once again, it may be considered essential to have at least two qualified dispensers if the pharmacy is to open six days a week.

Shop assistant

A shop assistant will only be required if it is the intention of the in-house pharmacy to sell a respectable quantity of retail goods. Local newspapers will provide a ready source of information on this score.

More details about employees will be found in Chapter 7.

Other recurring expenses

Care should be taken here that the new in-house pharmacy rent, 'rates', heating and lighting are not absorbed by the health centre. It is of course essential that the new business does rent its premises from the existing general practice business. A fair rent can be determined by consulting local businesses. Although this has been mentioned earlier, it is an expense and must be included.

All other services obtained from the host primary care practice will have to be paid for at current business rates.

Dispensing practice

The establishment of an in-house pharmacy will adversely affect the dispensing of an existing dispensing practice or any other dispensing practice nearby. The one-mile rule will apply and the practice will lose its dispensing rights to patients within the one-mile area. That is no reason not to go ahead in most cases. After all, some will be pre-empting a potential pharmacy application and far better to have your own pharmacy than lose the dispensing to an incomer.

Even a pharmacy that only breaks even may be better than losing income to another business.

However, there is another consideration – the Essential Small Pharmacy Scheme (ESPS). The new pharmacy may qualify for the ESPS (*see* p. 20). After all, there is nothing in the regulations to say that the medical practice must give up its dispensing rights to those of its patients outside the mile, simply to make the pharmacy viable.

Keep the two businesses clearly separate, as they are, and the pharmacy may qualify for this very useful subsidy if the PCO considers a pharmacy to be 'necessary or desirable' in the village. In that case the general practice will retain its dispensing income from patients outside the mile and the partners' pharmacy business will have income from dispensing within the mile plus the ESPS income. The dispensing practice may come to an arrangement with the pharmacy about dispensing for patients more than a mile from the pharmacy. In that way, the duplication of dispensing staff will be avoided.

Summary

Having read the preceding chapter and made a few enquiries it should be obvious to most that the pharmacy would be viable. If it is not profitable in its own right, then, assuming it is wanted by the NHS, then it will be made profitable through the ESPS subsidy.

So, what's stopping you? Let's get on with it.

References

1   Commons Health Committee (2003) *The Fifth Report of the Session 2002–03*. Stationery Office, London.
2   Department of Health (updated regularly) *The Drug Tariff*. Stationery Office, London.
3   *Chemist & Druggist Directory* (published annually by CMP Data & Information, Tonbridge).
4   *Medeconomics* (published monthly), Haymarket Medical Ltd, London.

Chapter 3

Getting on with it

Special considerations for dispensing practices

A special consideration for the dispensing practice that is considering opening a pharmacy is to pre-empt a pharmacy application. If this is the case, they should be on the alert for increases in their dispensing and practice population figures. After all, no one is in a better position than they to know whether a pharmacy application would be viable.

In the heady days of the then new 'loophole' several pharmacy owners put in abortive applications for quite small villages, more in hope than expectation, it seemed.

Dispensing practices should always be on the alert. If in doubt, nothing is to be lost by putting in an application. If it is rejected for the practice, it will also be rejected, under Clothier, for any pharmacy applicant for the next five years, unless there are 'significant' changes to the population density or the rurality of the area — subject, of course, to a loophole application. Generally speaking, there is no defence against 'loophole' applications other than being prepared.

However, one lawyer has suggested dispensing practices can take advantage of what he calls a 'sub-loophole'. Apparently, this indicates that where an applicant 'intends to provide pharmaceutical services in the place of, and at the same location as another person' the 'prejudice' clause does not apply. According to the solicitor, this means that a doctor, having formed a pharmacy company, would apply to replace his existing dispensary with a pharmacy and this application must be considered like that of a pharmacist already on the pharmaceutical list.

It is to be wondered whether this may be trumped by the fact that, according to the regulations, dispensing doctors do not provide 'pharmaceutical services' and therefore cannot fulfil that clause if it is rigidly applied to 'pharmaceutical services'.

The solicitor goes on to say that the doctor's company application must be prompt, but also says that if there are two or more applications they should only be considered in chronological order if there are no other deciding factors. A doctor with existing premises has a decided advantage if the application is prompt and would, possibly, have the company's application considered first.

That is another good reason to be well prepared along the lines suggested in this book.

An essential piece of advice all medical practices about to seek permission to have a pharmacy should heed is that it is common courtesy to consider their colleagues 'down the road'. Do any of them dispense to any part of the area that your new pharmacy will cover? If so, please invite them in for a discussion on what you are about to do.

The one-mile rule will apply to all doctors dispensing within a radius of one mile of your new pharmacy.

If the other practice will lose a significant amount of their dispensing, it may be that you can compensate them in some way? Once upon a time there was a compensation scheme where dispensing doctors compensated chemists whose businesses they had affected, and vice versa. Unfortunately, chemists were more successful at taking over doctor dispensing than doctors were the reverse, so the outflow from the chemists' fund became too great to sustain and this voluntary agreement was terminated.

You can do better than that, surely? Compensation could be either as a negotiated lump sum or an appropriate share in the business, perhaps.

Make the final decision

- Obtain copies of the legal requirements and regulations for pharmacies (*see* Chapter 4).
- Revise your understanding of Health & Safety and other regulations.
- Check for local dispensing practices.
- Check viability.
- Determine whether there is space for a pharmacy and other services in your premises.
- Draw up a rough plan indicating changes to premises or extensions.
- Possibly check outline plans with the Pharmaceutical Society for approval.
- Find a pharmacy designer (*see* Chapter 8).
- Obtain estimates for work to be done.
- Enquire about planning permission for change of use.
- Will the district valuer be interested?

Purchase a company, then:

- obtain copies of current application regulations and an application form
- alternatively, enquire about OFT-inspired changes in the regulations
- employ a solicitor experienced in pharmacy applications
- draw up and submit the application, if required.

If the application is successful:

- employ a superintendent pharmacist
- proceed to shopfitting, stocking, etc.

The final decision to go ahead

There is a great deal to be considered and considered carefully, apart from viability (*see* Chapter 2), before the final decision is made to go ahead with an application. None of the considerations should be rushed. Whatever may happen to the regulations, whether there is deregulation or not, if you own the premises, time will be on your side. Having said that, beware of the next door shop becoming vacant. Keep your ear to the ground. Are any of the local estate agents your patients?

Making the final decision to go ahead with an application

No decision can properly be reached without being conversant with the NHS regulations and the legal requirements the pharmacy company will have to work under. Many dispensing doctors may already know them. They include:

* Misuse of Drugs Act 1971
* Poisons Act 1972
* Medicines Acts, 1968 and 1971.

Then there are the laws regulating the sale of goods:

* Sale of Goods Act 1979
* Supply of Goods and Services Act 1982
* Intoxicating Substances (Supply) Act 1985
* Trade Descriptions Act 1968
* Consumer Credit Act 1974
* Consumer Protection Act 1987
* General Product Safety Regulations 1994
* Price Marking Order 1991
* Sunday Trading Act 1994.

Most GPs and their practice managers will be fully aware already of the current employment legislation, but just in case, it includes:

* Sex Discrimination Acts, 1975 and 1984
* Race Relations Act 1976
* Disability Discrimination Act 1995
* Working Time Directive 1998
* Health & Safety (Young Persons) Regulations 1997
* Health & Safety Regulations
* Asylum and Immigration Acts, 1996, 1999 and subsequent.

All the above will be described in some detail in the next chapter.

Checking the existing premises for space

Obviously there is little point going ahead with any thoughts for a pharmacy if there is no free space on the premises or if none can be created. A visit to a number of local pharmacies to check on the size of their dispensaries will give a fair impression of how much space will be needed. It is not as much as would be expected.

If in doubt, have a word with the RPSGB, which will have the final say on the adequacy of your premises.

While doing this think hard about the space required for a visiting dentist and optician. Both will be needed to satisfy *The NHS Plan*[1] definition of a one-stop primary care centre. This is best done after contacting members of those professions who may find a presence in your health centre an attractive proposition, if the rent is right.

Do bear in mind that although the optician and dentist may well be required to fulfil the definition of a one-stop health centre, it is the pharmacy that will provide the greater income, by far, so make the rent attractive. The supermarkets call such marketing 'loss-leading'.

The NHS Plan seems also to need a health visitor to be on the premises, but there are few practices that do not already have the services of this profession. Her room may possibly be shared with the social worker.

Drawing up rough plans

Planning the premises should perhaps be with the help of an architect, but there is a great deal to be said for the partners spending an evening or two playing with a plan of the building to get some idea of the possibilities.

Find out which walls are weight-bearing and which may be easily removed and where the various services run. Think about the convenience of access for the disabled. This has been a requirement since Spring 2004. Then consider access from both the street and from the health centre because the pharmacy may be open at times when the health centre is closed or vice versa.

Planners should always plan for ease of access for customers, including the disabled: therefore, the pharmacy should not be on either an upper floor or in a basement unless there is access by lift. The same applies to the room(s) rented to the visiting optician and dental practice.

Dispensing doctors have already asked whether the pharmacy should be physically separate from the existing dispensary. They need not be, but what is essential is that the two businesses are legally separate. There may be charges from one to the other to cover the services provided and, of course, rent for use of the practice premises should be paid by the pharmacy.

It is at this stage that thought may be given to building an extension to house one or more of the recommended professions. In the long term an extension is likely to be cost-effective, if the practice has sufficient land available without needing to eliminate too much car parking.

Estimates for alterations or extensions

Your architect may well be able to provide some indication of the expenses involved. These are essential before making your final decision and do not forget to include an amount for shopfitting, as mentioned in Chapters 2 and 8.

The architect may suggest three local building contractors who would be willing to give their estimates, even at this early stage. Do bear it in mind that shopfitting and equipping the pharmacy will add to the cost. The NPA provides an excellent service here (*see* Chapter 8).

Planning permission

It is no good accumulating all this information only to find that the local authority (LA) will refuse planning permission for change of use of part of the premises from a surgery to retail use. Have a quiet word with the LA planning department at an early stage. They should be able to give an indication of whether an application would be successful.

Plan your case carefully before that visit. Impress upon them that your company will be providing a service to the community and doing so according to government policy in *The NHS Plan.* Tell them of the additional services you will provide and how these will benefit patients far and wide. Ensure that they understand the difference between an in-house pharmacy and the high-street pharmacy – and all the advantages listed in Chapter 12.

When drawing up your plans always be aware of building regulations. All these and other considerations are described in Chapter 8.

Finally, the district valuer may be interested in the increased value of the premises. Be aware of that possibility, too.

Going ahead?

If you have collected all the above information then you will either have been completely put off the idea and everything with it or have been enthused to go ahead. For the sake of argument – and of continuing the book – it is assumed that you haven't been put off, so the next stage is to buy a company.

Company purchase is described in Chapter 5. It is very straightforward and inexpensive. It is not essential to employ a pharmacist at this stage.

The application regulations

If the OFT modifications are enacted then there may be no need for an application. Instead, a simple notification may be required together with an approval certificate, or similar document, from, say, the RPSGB. The PCO should be notified of the other 'one-stop' services provided on the premises. However, all that remains to be seen.

This chapter is relevant to current regulations and there will be many practices that could and should take advantage of those.

In the case of rural applications the Clothier Regulations must be followed, but as the practice will be applying against its own dispensing rights, there is no need to describe those regulations here. They are discussed in full in *The Complete Dispenser.*[2] The Control of Entry Regulations[3] and the application form are described in Chapter 6.

When you have read them it is time to engage the expert help of a solicitor familiar with, at least, NHS dispensing matters and, preferably, pharmacy applications. One such solicitor was mentioned in Chapter 1 and others are known to the author. A lot will depend upon his and your expertise in drawing up the formal application.

If the application is successful or not required, then will be the time to find a superintendent pharmacist to manage the business. Included in his duties will be the interviewing and appointment of other staff, among which the most important will be a second, part-time pharmacist and at least one qualified dispenser. None of these secondary appointments need be made until the premises are equipped and ready for occupation. All this is covered in Chapters 7 to 10.

References

1 Department of Health (2000) *The NHS Plan*. Stationery Office, London.
2 Roberts D (2002) *The Complete Dispenser* (4e). Communications International Group, London.
3 *The NHS (Pharmaceutical Services) Regulations 1992 (Control of Entry Regulations)*. Stationery Office, London.

Chapter 4

Preliminary steps: laws and regulations

The measures the practice can take to set the ball rolling before engaging an expensive solicitor will be found in this chapter. The NHS pharmacy regulations are discussed in some detail together with the mass of legal requirements for pharmacists and pharmacies.

The preliminary steps mainly consist of gathering and understanding information prior to the formal submission of an application, or a notification, should an application not be needed following the government's possible changes to the pharmacy entry regulations.

Two non-NHS bodies may be interested in your plans – the district valuer and the LA planning office.

The district valuer

Those who still have the old 'Red Book'[1] should turn to page 157, section 51.38 onwards, which deals with the review of payments made for premises owned by practitioners. Normally the review is three-yearly, but where there have been significant changes to the premises there must be a review of their suitability and a new rental value agreed.

Obviously, when premises are modified to allow an independent business to operate, significant changes will have been made and the value of the property changed. A fresh PREM 1 form should be submitted to the district valuer when the pharmacy has formally taken over its part. The district valuer will then assess the current market rent under the new circumstances.

There are then two possibilities.

Any part of the premises no longer used by the practice will be excluded from consideration. That, of course, would mean that the pharmacy part of the previous practice would be excluded and, therefore, the market valuation of the remainder will reduce. Not to worry, because the loss will largely be made up by the rent from the pharmacy.

Alternatively, the total value may have been increased because of the existence of the pharmacy.

At this preliminary stage, however, you need do nothing along these lines other than note that a new application will have to be made, so a new PREM 1 should be obtained and filed away in preparation. At the same time the cost rent regulations should be obtained and carefully read, together with details of changes made under the new GMS contract of 2004.[2]

A good source of information can be found at, www.redbook.i12.com/rb/Docs/rb898.htm together with the old Red Book 51.50.1 – 51.50.6.

It is important to remember that the district valuer is quite prepared to debate the figure arrived at – and so should you be.

The local authority

This body has a number of interests in what you are intending to do – planning, possibly building regulations and, finally, rent and 'rates'.

By opening a retail outlet such as a pharmacy the use of your building is being changed and planning permission will be required for the part of the building intended for use as the pharmacy. It pays to involve the planning officer at an early stage because he will have some knowledge as to whether such a change will be rejected out of hand.

It may seem unlikely that it would be, because a surgery or primary care centre should be well set up with parking spaces, the shortage of which has been a factor in the refusal of many an application by other businesses. The other consideration – the flow of traffic into and out of the premises is not likely to increase very much as most pharmacy customers will come from the surgery portion of the premises or on foot along the street. However, many surgeries are in listed buildings and that may prove to be troublesome.

Have a word in the planning officer's ear, even before formal plans are drawn up, but before doing so have a persuasive case ready. That case could include the benefits to the community in having a pharmacy on your premises, mentioning the government's *NHS Plan*.

At a much later stage, when the pharmacy is about to function, the local authority must be told of its existence in order to value it for local or business tax purposes. Don't forget, at the same time to have the remaining general practice premises revalued in case that tax will need to be reduced.

The primary care organisation

The PCO will need to be involved at this stage, also, for the purpose of adjusting the payment for the remaining general practice premises. Under the new GMS contract premises payments are not paid through the global sum but through separate arrangements. In England all premises funding will be held by a lead PCT within each strategic health authority (SHA). Paragraph 5.44 of *New GMS Contract 2003*,[2] page 41 states that:

> The existing SFA provisions for premises will be replaced. Under the new funding arrangements PCOs will have greater flexibility in funding premises to allow, for example, investment in premises to facilitate delivery of an extended range of primary medical services. Under the new contract there will be a system of rules which set minimum standards for new or refurbished buildings and guidance which offers support to PCOs on costs by setting benchmark costs rather than limits.

So it may be possible to receive some funding from the PCO for your improvements towards becoming a 'one-stop primary care centre'. That funding may not be for the alterations for a pharmacy, but it may help towards modifications to include the optician, dentist and health visitor. Be prepared to ask them at an early stage.

All this was in the 2003 new contract blue book which, we are all assured by the GPC, has not changed in any essential way since it was voted upon and accepted by GPs in 2003. The new document is not available at the time of writing this book, but it is necessary to caution doctors to examine the final presentation of the contract carefully because it has been changed, despite what the GPC says, in some very substantial ways.

The application

The formal application, under the existing regulations, will be covered fully in Chapter 6. At this stage it is only necessary to obtain a copy of the appropriate regulations and an application form. They are:

* *NHS (Pharmaceutical Services) Regulations 1992, No. 662 – Amendments to 1999*[3]
* *Application for Inclusion in a Pharmaceutical List – Schedule 3 Part 1.*[4]

Both documents are obtainable from the PCO or from The Stationery Office.

Hopefully, for many, if and when the OFT changes come into effect these documents will no longer be required. Instead some form of notification and premises approval mechanism will replace them.

Legal requirements for pharmacies and pharmacists

Please note here, that this author makes no pretence to be a solicitor nor any kind of expert on legal matters. It is essential that a qualified solicitor be consulted before taking action on any of the matters discussed below.

Pharmacy terms of service and the authority's duties

The NHS Terms of Service for a pharmacist are set out in Chapter 7, which relates to the staff of the dispensary. Included in the Terms of Service are:

* the regulations
* *The Drug Tariff*
* the disciplinary committee procedure
* the tribunal procedure
* an appeals procedure.

The authority – the PCO – has a legal duty to arrange for 'pharmaceutical services' for all NHS patients in its area when ordered by a doctor or a dentist.
By definition, as mentioned earlier, only pharmacists may provide pharmaceutical services.

The regulations are set out in: *NHS (Pharmaceutical Services) Regulations 1992,
No. 662.* There have been several subsequent amendments and all should be
requested from the PCO at an early stage in your considerations. The solicitor will
need them later.

'Pharmaceutical services' consist of the supply of drugs, medicines, appliances,
some supplemental services and contraceptive substances and appliances. These
services may be provided by pharmacists, pharmacy companies and appliance
contractors. As has been mentioned before, dispensing doctors do not provide
'pharmaceutical services' but they are allowed to dispense under limited circumstances according to the Clothier Regulations. As this is outside the remit of this
book it will not be discussed in more detail. Further information on doctor dispensing may be obtained from *The Complete Dispenser.*[5]

A pharmacist contracts his services to the authority and is, in the regulations,
referred to as 'the contractor'. The pharmacist's contract is, at the time of writing,
under just the same kind of thorough review as was the GP's in 2002–04. What
the outcome will be is unknown, so it is only possible to set out the essential
details of the current contract.

The contractor must:

• dispense all NHS prescriptions within a reasonable time
• keep certain minimum opening hours (this may become more detailed in the
  new pharmacy contract)
• abide by their Terms of Service as currently set out in Schedule 2 of the 1992
  Regulations.

Failure to abide by the Terms of Service will precipitate a disciplinary hearing.

Supervision

The NHS Regulations state: '5(1) Drugs shall be provided by or under the direct
supervision of a pharmacist.' The supervising pharmacist must be fit to engage in
pharmacy and not suspended from the Pharmaceutical Register.

The authority has a right to know the names of any registered pharmacist
employed for the provision of drugs from the pharmacy.

The service provided by the pharmacy

The service must be reasonably prompt, taking into account the scarcity of the
medicine and the urgency of the supply according to the patient's medical
condition. Any person who presents a valid, signed prescription form must,
without exception, be supplied, as above.

Any drug ordered by the prescriber must be dispensed as written on the signed
prescription form. There is no right to substitute generic for branded product.
If the pharmacist has doubts about a prescription he should contact the prescribing

doctor or dentist. Certain missing details, such as the quantity, strength or dose may be entered on the prescription by the pharmacist, using his judgement. Otherwise the drug must be supplied in a suitable container in the quantity ordered by the prescriber.

Original packs – patient packs – must be broken open if that was the obvious intention of the prescriber, otherwise complete packs may be dispensed. The pharmacy may dispense emergency supplies where the prescriber is known to the pharmacist and agrees to provide the signed form within three days. This does not apply to scheduled drugs (*see* below).

The supply of the wrong drug is a breach of the Terms of Service.

The pharmacy is required to make available to the authority records of any supplemental services such as patient medication records and residential home services, for which fees are claimed.

Any pharmacy may at any time apply, with three months notice, to be removed from the authority's list of pharmacies. The authority may agree to a shorter date or may itself ask for the removal of the pharmacy from the NHS list.

Pharmacies may provide a practice leaflet with details of their hours, services provided, alternative pharmacies out-of-hours, and a procedure for commenting on or complaining about the services provided.

Other duties of the pharmacist are described in Chapter 7.

Legal requirement applying to pharmacies

At the preliminary stage it is important that the partners are aware of the law as it affects pharmacy. The appropriate laws are:

- Misuse of Drugs Act 1971
- Poisons Act 1972
- Medicines Act, 1968 and 1971.

The retailing laws and regulations are:

- Sale of Goods Act 1979
- Supply of Goods and Services Act 1982
- Intoxicating Substances (Supply) Act 1985
- Trade Descriptions Act 1968
- Consumer Credit Act 1974
- Consumer Protection Act 1987
- General Product Safety Regulations 1994
- Price Marking Order 1991
- Sunday Trading Act 1994.

Then there is the plethora of employment regulations with which most practice managers will be familiar, if not the doctors.

- Sex Discrimination Acts, 1975 and 1984
- Race Relations Act 1976
- Disability Discrimination Act 1995
- Working Time Directive 1998
- Health & Safety (Young Persons) Regulations 1997

- Asylum and Immigration Acts, 1996, 1999 and subsequent
- Workplace (Health, Safety and Welfare) Regulations 1992, No. 3004.

All the above will be briefly described below in sufficient detail to give a taste of each Act or Regulation for information purposes only.

The Misuse of Drugs Act 1971

The Shipman Enquiry will almost certainly recommend extensive changes here and it will remain to be seen whether the government implements those recommendations.

The 1971 Act covers 'controlled or dangerous drugs' (CDs) and the 1985 Regulations provide five schedules with different degrees of control for the drugs included in each schedule.

Section 12 of the Act empowers the Home Secretary to prohibit a doctor, dentist or pharmacist convicted under the Act from dealing in CDs or even authorising their use. Section 23 authorises the police and others to enter premises such as pharmacies or surgeries to inspect CD stocks and paperwork.

The five schedules under the Regulations are:

- *Schedule 1*: The controls here are the strictest and the drugs included are those causing problems through social misuse such as LSD, raw opium, mescaline and many more. They are all listed. These drugs are prohibited from importation, exportation or possession without a licence from the Home Secretary. Cannabis has recently been rescheduled out of this list.
- *Schedule 2*: The medically useful CDs are included in this category. Morphine, pethidine, diamorphine and amphetamines are examples of the more than 100 drugs in the full list. There are strict controls about their possession, keeping, use and record keeping. Doctors and pharmacists may compound them. At present the doctor's prescription must be handwritten in full by the doctor, although there are moves to permit computer prescriptions under careful circumstances. A record of their use must be kept in a CD register.

  The Shipman Enquiry is likely to give detailed advice on the record keeping, storage and destruction of this group of drugs in an attempt to provide a foolproof audit trail.
- *Schedule 3*: Barbiturates, some appetite suppressants and pentazocine are included in this group. Records need not be kept in a CD register, but the pharmacist (or dispensing doctor) should retain purchase invoices.
- *Schedule 4*:
  - Part I: anabolic steroids
  - Part II: mainly the benzodiazepines other than temazepam.

  They are exempt from import/export restrictions and there are no restrictions on their possession as medicinal products only. Anabolic steroids are frequently traded in by sportsmen and their trainers. They are detectable after use.
- *Schedule 5*: Dilute preparations of Schedule 2 drugs are included here, such as weak preparations of codeine or morphine. Invoices must be kept by the pharmacist for two years.

Section 4 of the Act prohibits production of the drug other than by, among others on a carefully drawn up list, 'a pharmacist acting in his capacity as such'. The list of suppliers is equally carefully drawn up and, of course, includes pharmacists.

Unlawful possession of a CD is a criminal act, as is lawful possession with the intent to unlawfully supply.

Keeping CDs – CDs must be kept in a locked receptacle such as a safe, cabinet or room for which only the pharmacist has the key. The safe or cabinet must be secured to the floor or wall. The details of the construction of an approved safe are set out in the Act.

Dispensing a CD – A community pharmacist may only dispense a CD prescription if:

- the prescription is correctly handwritten by the prescriber (*see* below)
- the pharmacist knows and recognises the signature
- the pharmacist knows it to be genuine
- the prescriber's address is in the UK
- it is not post-dated
- it is not later than 13 weeks after the date on the prescription
- the prescription is dated with the date the drug is supplied
- the supply of that drug is then entered into a CD register.

Records for controlled drugs must be kept in a bound, not loose-leaf, register sectioned for each class of drug. Entries must be made in date order in indelible ink and made within 24 hours of dispensing or receipt.

The entry must contain the name and address of either the supplier or the patient and list the amount supplied with the form of the drug. Errors must not be obliterated, but simply lined through, asterisked with the correction listed as close to the original entry as possible. The register must be available for inspection by a police officer or other authorised person for two years after the last entry.

The prescription may only be dispensed (at present) if the following details are in the prescriber's handwriting:

- the name and address of the patient
- the dosage
- the strength and form of the drug – pill, capsule, etc
- the quantity prescribed – in words and figures
- the prescriber's signature.

Also on the prescription, but printed, must be the prescriber's name and address and the date of the prescription. Repeats are only permitted for Schedules 4 and 5 drugs.

The destruction of CDs by pharmacists – Although there is no requirement to keep records or have witnesses for the destruction of CDs returned by patients, it is good practice for a dated record containing details of the destruction to be made separately from the Drug Register. The RPSGB has a protocol for CD destruction:

> Following advice from a company dealing with pharmaceutical waste, the advice to use bleach when denaturing controlled drugs has now been revised. It is now recommended that hot, soapy water is used when destroying solid dose and parenteral formulations. Problems can arise if bleach is used in pharmaceutical waste as residual bleach mixes with chemicals used to clean bins if they are to be recycled and toxic fumes can be produced as a result.

Liquid formulations may be destroyed by mixing them with cat litter and Fentanyl patches should have the backing removed and the patch then should be folded upon itself. The Society then advises that the resultant mixture can be added to general pharmaceutical waste.

It is mandatory, according to the Regulations, that outdated, undispensed pharmacy stocks may only be destroyed in the presence of an authorised witness. Such witnesses include any serving police officer and Home Office inspectors, including certain medical and pharmaceutical advisors. It should be noted that PS inspectors will not, under normal circumstances, act as witnesses to CD destruction. A record of the destruction must be kept in the CD register.

Not all this advice is, of course, part of the Act. Further advice on the destruction of CDs is given in *The Complete Dispenser*[5] (q.v.).

The above are extracts of the most important sections of the Misuse of Drugs Act. There is a great deal more to it than shown. Pharmacy owners are advised to obtain and read the full Act.

The Poisons Act 1972

The Poisons Act defines poisons, deals with only non-medicinal poisons and sets out how they should be treated. Medicinal poisons are covered by The Medicines Act 1968. Recommendations about poisonous substances are made by the 16-person Poisons Board. It is of little, other than academic, interest to GPs, but pharmacists deal in poisons and, interestingly, may even sell them to doctors for professional use. The rules are detailed and enforced rigorously.

The Poisons List is in two parts:

1   Part I: those that may only be sold by a pharmacist
2   Part II: those that may be sold by pharmacists or listed sellers as permitted by local authorities.

It is enforced by the local authority and The Pharmaceutical Society.

Schedule 1 poisons include:

- strychnine
- arsenic
- fluoroascetic acid
- thallium salts
- zinc phosphide.

There are, in total, 12 schedules and all are listed in close detail.

The Poisons Rules for a pharmacy state that:

- all sales must be supervised by the pharmacist
- poisons must be stored separately away from the public and from food
- purchasers of Schedule 1 poisons must be known to be of good character or they must present a certificate from, for instance, the police saying they are of good character. Poisons cannot, therefore, be sold to any Tom, Dick or Harry who comes in off the street
- records must be kept of Schedule 1 sales in a poisons register. This must include the:

– date of sale
– name and address of purchaser
– name and address of the provider of the certificate
– name and quantity of the poison
– intended use of the poison.

The entry should be signed by the purchaser.

Not part of the Act, but it should be possible in these days of IT excellence to check that the purchaser's address actually exists.

Once again, the above does not completely describe the Act in question, but merely extracts 'the meat' from it. Obtain and become familiar with the Act.

The Medicines Act 1968

The Medicines Act 1968 is a very long and somewhat legalistic document that is difficult to penetrate. It was enacted as a response to the thalidomide tragedy and in advance of the UK's entry to the EEC.

One of the purposes of the Act was to form a Medicines Commission to advise ministers who have the responsibility for licensing medicines. Licensing is carried out by the Medicines Control Agency of the Department of Health which, for their part, are advised by the Committee on the Safety of Medicines.

Any new medicine, whether manufactured in the UK or imported, must have a product licence (PL), which must be displayed on the packaging of every packet sold, e.g. PL1234L. Parallel imports are shown as PL(PI) 1234M, for instance.

The Act details what may be considered as a medicinal product. It includes among the classifications, products which treat, prevent or diagnose diseases, produce anaesthesia or are contraceptive agents.

Other sections of the Act describe imported products and the advertising of medicines. The Act also details the labelling requirements.

It is the Medicines Act that gives permission for a qualified pharmacist to dispense defined medicines – as opposed to only OTC products. Briefly, a pharmacist may prepare or dispense a medicinal product only if it is done:

• in a registered pharmacy
• under the supervision of a pharmacist
• according to the instructions given by the purchaser
• if the product is to be administered by the purchaser to himself or as a carer.

Labelling and the Medicines Act – Full details of this are set down in the *Medicines (Labelling) Amendment Regulations 1976, 1977, 1978, 1992 and 1994.*

The pharmacist (or dispensing doctor) must ensure that the following five details are indelibly printed in English on every medicine dispensed:

1   the patient's name
2   the pharmacy's name and address
3   the date of dispensing
4   *Keep out of the reach of children* or a similar message
5   the quantity dispensed.

The Pharmaceutical Society will enforce these requirements.

Other details, recommended but not compulsory, are:

• the name of the drug
• the directions for use
• suggested precautions during use
• storage conditions
• expiry date
• warnings and/or side-effects.

Manufacturers are ordered to include a long list of other details on original pack outers, but they do not concern us here — fortunately.

It would be a brave pharmacist who removed any warning information provided by the manufacturer. More labelling advice is to be found in the *British National Formulary*.[6]

Control of the sales of medicines

The Medicines Act 1968, in various places, puts restrictions on who may sell medicines and where, as well as defining a medicine. Medicines are classified into three groups.

1 *Prescription only medicines (POM)* — These may only be supplied from a pharmacy under the supervision of a pharmacist after being prescribed by a doctor, dentist or vet. In recent years a gaggle of others have been granted prescribing rights to certain drugs, e.g. pharmacists and nurses.
2 *Pharmacy medicines (P)* — These may only be sold in a pharmacy under the supervision of a pharmacist. A doctor's prescription is not required.
3 *General sales list (GSL)* — GSL medicines must be sold from a lock-up shop rather than a market stall, for instance, but it is unnecessary for it to be a pharmacy or for there to be a pharmacist present.

The Medicines Act 1968 goes on to define a prescription in detail. It exonerates a pharmacist who, in good faith, dispenses a prescription according to the prescriber's instructions, even if those instructions are subsequently found to be incorrect. We all know that there are exceptions to this where the pharmacist should have known better and thus to contact the prescriber. The pharmacist will be judged by the assumed actions of his contemporary peers.

Many details of the prescription must be recorded and kept for two years. The details required are listed in the Act.

Prescriptions can be faxed to the pharmacy, if urgent, but the original must be sent as soon as practicable. The Act does not demand that the original should be with the pharmacist at the time of dispensing. Schedules 2 and 3 medicines, as controlled drugs, are an exception. The prescription for these must be at the pharmacy at the time of dispensing.

The Act describes supervision and retail staff. This will be covered in Chapter 7.

The wholesaling of medicines is thoroughly covered by the Act together with a list of who may buy medicines. This may be important to your pharmacy as you may wish to supply your dispensing practice. Basically, the regulations are that the pharmacy would be wholesaling if:

- its wholesaler sells to the pharmacy, which then sells the medicine over the counter
- its wholesaler sells to the pharmacy, which then sells it to a doctor who administers it.

It is not wholesaling if:

- its wholesaler sells to the pharmacy, which then *gives* it to a doctor who administers it.

This may be of interest to one or two dispensing practices that have previously been advised otherwise.

Parallel imports – By definition these are imported from other member states of the EU and may have been made in the UK. They are called 'parallel imports' because they are sold in parallel with the UK manufactured items, but not, usually, by the manufacturer, which may be quite upset by their sale.

They are of advantage to pharmacists because there may be a marked price difference between the UK and the other EU country versions of the identical product.

The EU bans the restriction of such imports if:

- the import is therapeutically equivalent to the UK product
- manufacturing standards are correct
- it is manufactured by the same group of companies or under licence from them.

The parallel imported medicine must:

- be labelled in English or have an English label substituted for the original
- have the same brand name as the English version.

Collection and delivery schemes – The Medicines (Collection and Delivery Arrangements – Exemption) Order 1978, No. 1421 permit these schemes if:

- they are in accordance with a doctor's prescription
- the supply is under a pharmacy scheme
- the medicine is for human use.

The scheme allows chemists and dispensing doctors to use rural 'drop-off' points such as post offices, shops and the homes of trusted members of the public.

There is another delivery scheme that involves the collection of the prescription by the pharmacist from the doctor and the delivery of the medicine to the patient's house. In this case the pharmacist must have written consent from the patient and must use his professional judgement as to whether he should have a consultation with the patient about the medicine.

Finally, in the Medicines Act section, a pharmacist may dispense an urgent drug at the request of a doctor over the telephone and without the written prescription being to hand. The doctor must supply the script as soon as practicable.

There have been numerous Amendments or companion Acts over the years. These cover such topics as:

- the EU demand for product leaflets with each item
- a list of exempt herbal remedies
- the fluted bottles regulations
- intrauterine contraceptive devices
- contact lens fluids
- a chiropodist's list of preparations
- various veterinary preparations amendments
- a homoeopathic medicines advisory board
- the advertising and regulation of advertising of medicines.

The above is but a fraction of the whole. A couple of useful reference works are listed at the end of the book.

Retailing laws

The Sale of Goods Act 1979

Few doctors will have much knowledge of this Act and as they may well be seriously thinking of becoming part of a retailing venture it would be as well to know the gist of it.

Once again, what follows is guidance only and an experienced, qualified solicitor should be consulted before any action is taken.

The main provisions of the Act are:

- the seller must have the right to sell the goods
- the seller must pass on 'good title'
- if the seller is aware of, and passes on, details of defects the buyer takes his chances
- the goods must be as described on the package or by the salesman, otherwise payment must be refunded
- the goods must be of 'satisfactory quality'; 'you get what you pay for'
- the sale must be in the course of business
- buyers cannot reject faulty goods after purchase if the faults were shown before purchase
- if the buyer examines faulty goods before purchase he loses the right for compensation if he ought to have found the faults
- goods must be fit for the purpose for which they are sold.

Section 14(3) may well affect pharmacists. It says:

> Where the buyer sells the goods in the course of a business and the buyer ... makes known to the seller ... any particular purpose for which the goods are being bought, there is an implied condition that the goods supplied under the contract are reasonably fit for the purpose, whether or not that is a purpose for which such goods are normally supplied.

A very crude example would be if the pharmacist deliberately sold a 'cold' remedy for the treatment of indigestion while telling the customer it would be effective for that purpose. 'Cold' remedies are not licensed for such a purpose.

The Supply of Goods and Services Act 1982

This Act covers goods obtained in ways other than purchase, hire purchase or the use of trading stamps such as Air Miles. Services supplied and materials provided as a part of that service must be of 'satisfactory' quality in a similar way to The Sale of Goods Act. In pharmacy this would mean that, under Section 13 of the Act, a pharmacist would be caught out if he failed to take reasonable care while mixing and dispensing a prescription for a patient.

Other interesting sections provide for the completion of a service within a reasonable time and, if a price is not stated, that the customer will pay a 'reasonable' price.

The Intoxicating Substances (Supply) Act

More than likely your pharmacy will not be selling alcohol to its customers in order to help them pass the time while they are waiting. This Act, however, has nothing to do with that, but does make illegal the sale to minors of any substances that could be used for glue sniffing, for instance. The penalty is either six months in jail or a £5000 fine.

The Trade Descriptions Act 1968

The purpose of this Act is to prevent misleading or false descriptions being deliberately applied to goods. It is an offence to do so.

It may not be well known but the Act applies to the provision of services where the provider makes a materially false statement about:

- the nature of the service
- the approval or evaluation of the service
- the location of the service.

Pharmacists should be very, very careful when:

- labelling items for sale
- describing any service which they may be providing.

They should not act outside their area of expertise and imply that their advice is, for instance, an equivalent to that of a qualified medical practitioner.

The Consumer Credit Act 1974

The Consumer Credit Act is primarily concerned with, as it says, credit where the credit does not exceed £15 000. It attempts to ensure that advertisements are accurate. People accepting hire purchase or credit transactions must have full documentation about the transaction and must be given a cooling-off period for agreements made off business premises.

Some businesses need licences, of which there are six categories and any pharmacist offering delayed payment, staged payments or the loan of money in a transaction of less than £15 000 will need a licence. An exception arises when the retailer accepts no money 'upfront', but does allow the customer to pay in full at the end of a set time. In this case no licence is required.

Pharmacists may need a licence if they hire out surgical appliances, wheelchairs or other goods with a value of less than £15 000 for more than three months.

If a pharmacist introduces a customer to a finance company for the purpose of buying an expensive item such as an item of equipment, then he may need a licence for that, too – this time as a credit broker.

Further enquiries may be made of: Customer Credit Licensing Branch, Office of Fair Trading, Government Buildings, Bromyard Avenue, Acton, London, W3 7BB.

The Consumer Protection Act 1987

This interesting and important Act was the source of some minor disagreement of interpretation between the professions of pharmacy and medicine, so far as product liability is concerned.

The advice of the Medical Defence Union (MDU) in their booklet *Product Liability* is that records of each transaction must be made and kept. The NPA, on the other hand, disagreed, saying it was a waste of time.

This author comes down very firmly on the side of the MDU, especially so far as dispensing doctors are concerned. Sooner or later in this compensation-ridden age there will be a test case and the lack of proper records will hinder that case and, perhaps, be the reason for the chemist or doctor having huge amounts of compensation awarded against them.

As both dispensing doctors and pharmacists carry out a very similar, if not identical, action in dispensing it seems logical that pharmacists should also keep records. But they don't.

Under the Consumer Protection Act (CPA), following an EU Directive, any person injured by a defective product can sue the manufacturer for compensation, whether or not that manufacturer was negligent. The complainant must be able to prove:

- the product to be defective
- that he suffered damage of some sort
- that the damage was caused by the defective product
- that the defendant was the 'manufacturer' or was selling under an 'own brand' label.

Any pharmacist who mixes medicines extemporaneously is, by definition, the manufacturer. Any pharmacist who dilutes medicines not under written guidance from the original producer is the manufacturer. Any pharmacist who sells cough mixtures, for instance, under his own label, is the manufacturer. And the pharmacist will be liable under the product liability regulations if any patient or customer comes to harm through those products. The pharmacist will not be able to pass that responsibility down the chain. The term 'products' includes dressings, appliances, instruments or anything sold.

Any pharmacist who cannot provide the source of any product he sells or dispenses will, by default, become the manufacturer under this legislation. And that could be expensive if no records have been kept.

The MDU says:

> The clinical notes must show the basic information. In addition, it is important to be able to trace back from each dispensed prescription to the supplier or producer of the product. ('Product Liability', MDU, 1989)[7]

They recommend that record be kept of:

- the name and address of the patient
- the date of the transaction
- the name of the drug or product
- the dosage
- the frequency of dosage
- the quantity provided.

It is also useful to keep the batch number and expiry date. The record should be dated, signed and kept for 11 years.

There are other causes for liability:

- the obscuring of the manufacturer's instructions with the pharmacy label
- the mixing of two batches of the same drug in one container
- the (prohibited) reissue of returned stock.

If for medicine why not for pharmacy? The reader will need to make his own mind up about that.

The original DDA (1984–97) provided useful record cards for dispensing doctors. Unfortunately the new DDA Ltd discontinued them.

The General Product Safety Regulations 1994

The regulations state that goods sold must be safe under normal foreseeable conditions of use and must present either none or a minimal risk during use. The presence of the EU mark, CE, is sufficient proof unless the retailer has split a pack and does not pass on the maker's instructions with each portion.

Beware, the pharmacist who splits an original pack therefore becomes the producer as under the Consumer Protection Act, above.

The Price Marking Order 1991

Once again this is a regulation following an EU Directive. All goods sold on retail premises must have their price indicated in some way so that the customer can understand it. There may be future changes to this Order.

Sunday Trading Act 1994

The Sunday Trading Act permits small shops with a floor area of no more than 280 square metres, approximately 17 m square, to open on Sundays without restriction. Most in-house pharmacies will fall into this category and could well remain open to catch Sunday trade as well as to dispense medicines. However, retail pharmacies are exempt from this law so long as they do not sell products other than medicines.

The employment laws

This book is primarily directed at general medical practitioners who, by definition, may well employ a large staff. They will, of course, with their practice managers already be very familiar with all the following legislation, but no such publication would be complete without it.

The more detailed matters of the contract of employment, wages, redundancy, sick pay and other matters will be covered in Chapter 7. Details of more specific Acts follow below. It would be as well to pay great heed to them because many employers have fallen foul of one or the other and paid a heavy price for doing so.

The Employment Act 2003

This Act applies to all employers regardless of the number of employees and is designed to be family-friendly. Amongst its measures are:

* increasing maternity pay and maternity leave
* paternity leave
* adoptive parents' leave.

Maternity pay will shortly rise from £75 to £100 per week and leave to a year, 26 weeks of it being statutory maternity leave paid by the employer at a stated rate.

Fathers will be paid paternity leave if they have been employed for more than one year and parents who have adopted a child will also be entitled to some 'bonding' leave. However, the employers do have some rights as study of the Act will show.

The Act also carries some modifications to the grievance procedures. There are now three stages.

1   The employer must set out in writing why consideration is being given to disciplinary action and invite the affected employee to a meeting.
2   At the meeting the decision should be given to the employee with a right of appeal.
3   If there is an appeal there must be a further meeting and the employee must be informed of the outcome.

The Sex Discrimination Acts, 1975 and 1984

These Acts prevent employers from discriminating between men and women or between the married and single in matters of:

* recruitment
* terms and conditions of employment
* training
* promotion
* dismissal
* employee benefits.

There are some exceptions:

* women during pregnancy and childbirth
* where the special characteristic of the job makes it suitable for one sex or the other
* where in the previous year there were few or no members of that sex in a particular employment
* in specified professions such as the police or prison service.

It is unlawful to advertise in a way which could reasonably be taken as displaying an intention to offend against the Act. It is also unlawful to publish such an advertisement. This means that:

- specifying a particular sex is unlawful (exceptions are listed above)
- specifying conditions that would imply the job is suitable for one sex when, in fact, it is suitable for both.

Discrimination may be in one of two categories.

1 *Direct discrimination* occurs when there is less favourable treatment on the grounds of sex or marital status. A direct comparison between the sexes in the same employment must be shown.
2 *Indirect discrimination* against a woman occurs if the employer applies to her a requirement:
    - that would be applied to a man, but which few women can do
    - that cannot be justified
    - that is to her detriment, because she is unable to comply with it.

An extreme example would be where a height of 6 feet 4 inches was demanded for a caretaker.

The Equal Opportunities Commission administers and reviews the Act.

The Race Relations Act 1976
Direct or indirect racial discrimination is prohibited under this Act.

- *Direct discrimination* occurs when a person is treated less favourably due to their race.
- *Indirect discrimination* occurs if obstacles relating to race are put in place as terms of employment or the employee is victimised due to their race.

The term 'race' covers colour, race, ethnic or national origins and nationality. The phrase 'no black Irishmen need apply' would be another extreme example. It is unlawful to induce others to discriminate.

The Commission for Racial Equality (CRE) advises and assists victims of racial discrimination and is very vigilant.

The Disability Discrimination Act 1995
This Act has the same effect for the disabled as the previous two do for sex and race discrimination.

'Disabled' includes individuals who for the foreseeable future (12 months) will have a disability. In other words, the disability need not be permanent. It covers both mental and physical disability, which may have the effect, long term, of substantially impairing a person's ability to carry on normal day-to-day activities.

Employers must take reasonable steps not to discriminate against disabled applicants during recruitment. The installation of ramps, the use of Braille and similar measures should be considered.

As there have been few cases under this Act it is strongly advised that if the pharmacy becomes involved in this area of litigation legal advice be sought at an early stage.

From 2004 all shops and public premises should have made reasonable adjustments to their premises to comply with the Act. The changes could involve the provision of:

* improved wheelchair access
* wide aisles between counters and shelving
* clear signs and good lighting
* loop systems for the hard of hearing
* easier access to counters.

Improved wheelchair access could simply be a bell on the outside of the building to alert helpful staff, rather than a ramp. However, ramps are possibly better.

The effect of the European Union on pharmacy

I wonder just how many of us fully understand the mechanism of the European Union, and how it affects us all and, of course, pharmacy?

There are five institutions covering law-making and implementation in the EU:

* Council of Ministers
* European Commission
* European Parliament
* European Court of Justice
* Economic and Social Committee.

The Council of Ministers consists usually of the foreign ministers of member countries and is, theoretically, the decision-making body. Potential laws come before the Council for discussion.

The European Commission consists of 17 commissioners plus an enormous number of helpers organised into Directorates-General. As a whole the Commission plans policy, mediates between governments and prosecutes those who break rules and treaties.

The European Parliament appears to be a talking shop with little power other than, to some extent, control the budget and pass opinion on ideas from the Commission.

The European Court of Justice interprets and applies community laws. Cases may be brought before it by countries or even individuals. It can impose fines on nations as well as individuals.

The Economic and Social Committee consists of interest groups appointed by Council to advise on economic matters.

European laws

European Regulations are mandatory on every country within the Union. Directives are also mandatory, but need legislation in member countries to enact them. They then override national laws.

The Working Time Directive

An introduction from Europe, this law covers the maximum duration of the working week, the leave entitlement, off-duty periods and rest periods. There are exceptions to it, but pharmacy staff are not among those, so become familiar with the legislation.

The Health & Safety (Young Persons) Regulations 1997

Once again this has been inherited from the EC. It sets clearer limits on the working life of young people under 18 years. To some extent it sets out the limits of such individuals' work. This has been assessed by their lack of experience and awareness of risks. The employer is required to make parents and young employees aware of the outcome of risk assessments and preventive measures taken to avoid those risks.

Other pharmacy-related directives

- *Directive 65/65/EEC* defines a medicinal product as one presented for treating or preventing disease or used with a view to making a medical diagnosis or restoring, correcting or modifying physiological functions – in humans or animals.
- *Directive 89/341/EEC* demands the supply of patient information leaflets.

There are other directives which entitle appropriately qualified pharmacists to work in any EU state. This is subject to linguistic ability. The qualifications are listed in yet another directive. Disqualification in one state disqualifies in all.

The Asylum and Immigration Act

Any observer of the daily papers will know that changes to this Act come almost weekly, so good advice is to seek help from a lawyer if in any doubt.

From the employer's point of view the Act makes it a requirement to make reasonable checks as to whether an employee or applicant is allowed to work in Britain. Failure to do so may result in large fines.

Dismissal of an employee

Most of the above has covered the employment of workers but, at some time or other, there may come the unpleasant and potentially dangerous task of having to dismiss an employee. There are very strict ways of going about this if an Employment Tribunal is to be avoided.

The simple way would be to give notice of termination in accordance with the contract of employment, assuming there is a set period mentioned in the contract. If there is not, then the courts will determine what a 'reasonable' period would be. Even if this is carried out there may still be a successful claim for compensation.

A fairly acceptable table of 'reasonable' periods would be:

- continuous employment between 1 week and 2 years – 1 week's notice
- over 2 years' continuous employment – 1 week for every year.

Summary dismissal

Summary dismissal, without notice and justification, is unlawful and damages may be brought for breach of contract or a case may be brought before an Industrial

Tribunal (IT). Breach of confidence by a member of staff in a doctor's surgery or a pharmacy may well be justification, especially if it has been detailed at interview and in the contract of employment.

If placed in such a situation then do not 'blow your top'; instead count to 10, explain to the employee that you are concerned and that you will be taking advice about the matter, then consult your solicitor urgently and listen carefully to what he has to say.

The next step would be to invite your employee to a meeting with you at an opportune time after consulting the solicitor.

Wrongful dismissal

As implied above, an employee alleging this may bring a civil case for wages lost through insufficient notice. The amount of compensation will be reduced to allow for:

- wages paid by another employer during the dismissal period
- tax and national insurance contributions from the wages
- benefits received from the state, e.g. unemployment benefit.

Unfair dismissal

Cases alleging unfair dismissal are very common in Industrial Tribunals under Section 94 of the Employment Rights Act 1996 because every employee has the right not to be unfairly dismissed.

For the case to succeed the employee must prove dismissal or constructive dismissal. Constructive dismissal occurs when the employer makes the employee's working life so intolerable that he resigns or simply leaves.

The employee must then prove unfairness and it is for the employer to give reasons for the dismissal. All reasonableness may be justified on the grounds of the employee's:

- lack of capability or qualifications
- misconduct. Only serious misconduct would justify immediate dismissal
- redundancy. This must be proven to be genuine and fair
- illegality to continue in the employment. A struck-off pharmacist, for instance could not continue to be employed as a pharmacist in a pharmacy.

Pregnancy and trade-union membership are rarely considered to be fair reasons for dismissal.

Industrial tribunal procedure

The employee must complain to the tribunal within three months of the dismissal and the employer must respond to notification of the complaint by the tribunal, within two weeks of the notification. There will then be an attempt by the Advisory, Conciliation, and Arbitration Service (ACAS) to resolve the matter 'out of court'.

The tribunal has the power to allow a successful applicant to be either reinstated or engaged in a similar job under the same employer. There may also be compensation awarded against the employer.

Where reinstatement is not appropriate, then compensation will be awarded according to a scale. There is no upper limit in unfair dismissal cases where dismissal is due to discrimination under EU legislation for equal pay, etc.

Redundancy

Employees cannot claim compensation awards for redundancy if they are:

* less than 2 years into employment
* over retirement age
* under 18 years of age
* on fixed-term contracts of greater than 2 years, but have signed away redundancy rights
* normally employed outside Britain.

It is possibly unlikely that any pharmacy employee will be made redundant, so greater detail on this legislation should be sought from your solicitor if required.

Summary

Ensure that this and all the other employment legislation is well understood by all interview panel members before drawing up advertisements, shortlists or interviewing candidates.

The interview panel should particularly beware of the effect of the amended Data Protection Act, which permits candidates access to any written notes made about them during the actual interview. Should there be anything apparently discriminatory, then the notes may be used in evidence during an employment tribunal or other case under one of the Acts described above. Any internal hieroglyphics will have to be translated, so any comments must be accurate, justifiable and polite.

It is not unknown for failed applicants to seek redress from Employment Tribunals, so get everything right at the start.

An employer's duties to the staff

In his excellent book, *Quality in the New GP Contract*, Dr Andrew Spooner[8] strongly recommends that the motivation of the staff will help get the best out of them. He suggests:

* annual appraisals
* written terms and conditions

- compliance with all statutory minimum employment rights and anti-discrimination laws
- compliance with the Health & Safety legislation
- a manual of staff employment practices such as bullying, sickness, absence, etc with comments
- job descriptions
- policies to prevent fraud and to protect staff income and pensions.

All these have been described earlier in this chapter but it is useful to have them drawn together in this way.

The Workplace (Health, Safety & Welfare) Regulations 1992

These Regulations apply to every workplace unless it be on a ship or related to building, engineering or mineral extractions. They require every employer to comply and that any modification of the workplace complies.

They are all-embracing Regulations, covering every aspect of the workplace including, briefly:

- *Maintenance* – all equipment must be clean and well maintained.
- *Ventilation* – every workplace must be well ventilated with fresh air and the ventilator must be fitted with a failure warning.
- *Temperature* – 'During working hours the temperature shall be reasonable'.
- *Lighting* must be sufficient and preferably natural light, if possible.
- *Cleanliness and waste materials* everywhere must be kept sufficiently clean and there must be no build-up of waste.
- *Workstations and seating* seating must be suitable and a footrest be provided if necessary. Precautions must be taken to avoid 'slips or falls'.
- *Conditions of floors and traffic routes* – floors must be suitable for the purpose. They must not be slippery or have holes and must be free of obstructions.
- *Falls or falling objects* – as far as is reasonably practicable measures must be taken to avoid these.
- *Windows* – it must be possible to open windows that are meant to be opened without danger and no open window must expose the employee to danger.
- *Window cleaning* – it must be possible to clean windows safely.
- *Organisation of traffic routes* – pedestrians must be able to circulate in safety. In a pharmacy this includes customers and staff.
- *Doors and gates* must be suitably constructed and safely installed.
- *Toilets* must be provided at readily accessible places, be well ventilated, clean and lit.
- *Washing facilities* must be suitable and sufficient.
- *Drinking water* must be provided for all persons, with cups.
- *Accommodation for clothing* this must be provided both for outdoor and any work clothing.
- *Facilities for changing* must be provided separately for men and women.
- *Rest facilities* – a suitable place must be provided for rest and eating.

Summary

What I have attempted to do in this chapter is to indicate some of the intricacies and dangers of the law and the perils of 'doing it yourself'. In all cases take advice from a legal expert.

Please note that I am taking that advice myself by repeating the above disclaimer!

Contracts of employment and related matters are covered in Chapter 7.

References

1   Department of Health. *General Medical Services: Statement of Fees and Allowances*. Stationery Office, London.
2   Department of Health (2003) *New GMS Contract*. Stationery Office, London.
3   *The NHS (Pharmaceutical Services) Regulations 1992, No. 662. Amendments to 1999 (Control of Entry) Regulations*. Stationery Office, London.
4   *Application for Inclusion in a Pharmaceutical List − Schedule 3 Part 1*. Stationery Office, London.
5   Roberts D (2002) *The Complete Dispenser*. Communications International Group, London.
6   *British National Formulary*. BMA and RPSGB, London. Regular updates.
7   Medical Defence Union (1989) *Product Liability*. MDU, London.
8   Spooner A (2004) *Quality in the New GP Contract*. Radcliffe Medical Press, Oxford.

Chapter 5

Forming your company

The next stage of getting on with it is to form your own company. This is essential because the only legal way a medical practice can provide routine medicines for their patients, other than from a doctor's emergency bag at night, is if the practice is a dispensing practice.

There may well be limited changes to this in the near future when out-of-hours doctors and possibly others will be permitted to provide full packs of emergency drugs on prescription and be paid for them by the NHS. But for the time being, there is strict separation between the professions according to the NHS maxim: 'The doctor shall prescribe and the chemist shall dispense, each according to their own special area of expertise.' The one exception is that pharmacists will shortly be allowed to prescribe from their own list of drugs.

It is possible that the entreaty of *The NHS Plan*, which promised to 'shatter the old demarcations which slowed down care' will eventually blur the margins sufficiently to allow more practices to dispense for their patients. Maybe this is a reason for the government's delay in implementing the DDA Ltd and GPC's proposals to ring-fence dispensing practices by actively preventing more practices from providing this valuable service to their patients.

The current measures to be taken to become a dispensing doctor are outside the remit of this book, but it is rewarding to the author that, for the time being, the number of these is still increasing year by year. That is unlikely to continue if the regulation changes proposed by the DDA Ltd and GPC, with the eager help of pharmacy, actually come to pass.

All about companies – well, nearly all

Remember that this book is a guide to the subject and that expert advice should be obtained from an experienced solicitor.

At this stage it would be as well to know a little about companies and company law. After all, you will be bound by it after setting up your company and not many of us are even slightly conversant with the relevant laws and regulations.

Limited companies are of three types:

- private limited company
- public limited company
- company limited by guarantee.

A *private limited company* will usually be small, with limited share capital. The structure is similar to that of a public limited company and will be described later in this chapter as being the type of company doctors may wish to set up for their own pharmacy.

A *public limited company*, otherwise known as a 'plc' needs to have share capital of more than £50 000. Plc shares may be offered to the public and may, but do not need to be, quoted on the stock exchange and sold through stockbrokers. Their structure is basically the same as that of the private limited company. It is unlikely that you are about to set out on such a venture except in the largest of primary care health centres.

If you attended a public school then the school was probably a *company by guarantee*, being a non-profit-making business. Religious and charitable organisations may also fall into this class. Pharmacies will not.

Benefits of a private limited company

The most important of these by a short head is that doctors generally cannot dispense to their NHS patients, but a company owned by doctors may do so simply because, in law, the company is a separate entity.

Some other benefits accruing from a private limited company are:

- its name is registered at Company House and is unique
- the value of their shares limits the liability of the shareholders
- money may be borrowed more readily
- there may be tax advantages
- employees may own shares, if available.

Being a separate legal entity a company can:

- carry out its own transactions
- sue or be sued (the shareholders have a limited liability)
- buy property

all in the name of the company. On the other hand, individual members of a company cannot sue for damages committed against the company.

There are a number of occasions where the separate entity rule does not apply and some of them may, at some time, be relevant to a pharmacy company of the type discussed here.

There are exceptions.

- If there are fewer than two board members for more than six months before the company ceases to trade, then the last member is liable together with the company for any debts incurred during the final six months.
- Undischarged bankrupts are liable for company debts while they are directors.
- You cannot start a new company with the same or similar name less than twelve months after the first company became insolvent.
- Companies cannot trade with fraudulent intent while being wound up.
- A director who should have known that a company, during winding up, would become insolvent becomes liable for some of the company's debts.
- Companies must not be formed simply to avoid tax.

The above merely gives the outline in each case. The detail can be supplied by a company solicitor.

Liability

It has already been mentioned that the term limited liability means that any single director or shareholder is financially liable only to the full value of the shares he holds. The fact that he may not have fully paid for them is not relevant. He would still be liable for their full value.

When a liquidator winds up a company he first realises all the assets of the company, if he cannot find a purchaser for it as a going concern. Should there not be sufficient funds after doing this then the next step would be to call on the shareholders. They would be liable as mentioned above.

Your company's name

No two companies can trade under an identical name. This is set down in the Companies Act 1985. The office of the Registrar of Companies has been set up specifically to examine all proposed names to prevent this happening. If it is noticed that two names are very similar then the more recent will be required to change its name within 12 months.

Money matters

All companies need money to function and in the majority of cases this is provided by the share capital. There are two kinds of shares. Ordinary and preference.

Ordinary shares are the most common. They usually have voting rights at company meetings and, of course, entitle the shareholder to a 'share' of the company profits, otherwise known as the dividend. The dividend paid at any one time is variable, both upwards and downwards, as several television advertisements have indicated in small print at the bottom of the screen. This has some advantages as will be seen below.

Although ordinary shares carry a greater risk, they also carry with them great benefits other than possible financial ones. It is from the group of ordinary shareholders that directors come and, therefore, they who decide how the company shall be run.

The shareholders in the small pharmacy company being described here will very probably be the partners in the practice and whoever else you choose to help finance the firm and benefit from it.

The term *preference shares* means what it says. These shareholders have priority over ordinary shareholders when the dividend is paid and a similar priority, to the value of their shares, if there are any assets left on winding up a company. However, the downside is that the dividend is usually at a fixed rate and that rate may, from time to time, be less than that paid to the ordinary shareholder. Another disadvantage is that, after a winding-up and after all shares have been repaid, if there are still any assets left over, the ordinary shareholders will be the beneficiaries not the preference shareholders.

Loan capital is another way of financing the company, but it is unlikely that your company will meet the need for this unless you allow ambition to run away with you. Suffice to say here that it involves mortgages, debenture stock and loan stock.

Colleagues involved in stock-exchange deals or other financial dealings may well already know the meaning of these terms. Most of us don't need to know. However, we are all familiar with mortgages.

Debenture stock usually has a fixed interest rate and is redeemed at a fixed date in the future. During winding-up periods they carry a similar priority to preference shares in the repayment of their interest and capital. Holders of debenture stock have no rights to vote or take any part in company matters.

Loan capital is commonly obtained from banks and is secured by a charge on the assets of the company, such as property or stock.

Other legal requirements

All companies must have:

- a registered office
- company stationery
- accounts
- a company seal and register
- company shareholders' meetings
- published annual returns
- prepared tax returns.

The registered office
It may surprise some people, but the registered office does not need to be the place of business — in this case — the pharmacy. It may be anywhere, but wherever it is, a company name must be prominently displayed as one should be at the place of business. That, of course, is not a problem with a pharmacy.

The tax inspector will deal with company matters at the registered company address, not at the pharmacy, unless the two are identical.

Company stationery
There are strict rules about company stationery and that includes notepaper, cheques, invoices and receipts. In every case the company name must appear and, in the case of letters, whether they be on notepaper, fax messages or emails, the registered address, place of registration and the registration number of the company must also be shown.

Accounts
Within six months of incorporation the company must ask for Form G224 to notify the registrar of the date for the presentation of the accounts. The accounts must be written to show clearly company:

- income and expenses
- assets and liabilities
- stock levels
- creditors and debtors.

The accounts must be audited by a certified accountant before the first annual general meeting (AGM) and presented at that meeting to shareholders. In the case of the small, in-house pharmacy owned by the doctors, this still applies although the event will be a much smaller affair. There may be no necessity for a separate auditor as the accountant would be acceptable.

Company seal and books

It does seem to be a little anachronistic, but there is still a legal requirement for a company seal for use on formal documents such as share certificates. The seal should be engraved with the company name. It does add a touch of interest to the proceedings, but I have heard it said that this rule is not strictly policed.

Registered books are required to list details of:

* shares of all kinds including debentures
* shareholders
* the issuing and transference of shares
* the directors and their interests
* the company secretary.

The minutes of company meetings should be kept in a separate book.

Company meetings

Board meetings are used for the running of the business and to ensure that the statutory requirements as listed above are being properly carried out.

General meetings are occasions when shareholders express their opinions about the running of the company, pass resolutions for changes and vote upon members of the board of directors. The first AGM must be within 18 months of the founding incorporation of the company.

At each AGM the directors of a company must:

* present the audited accounts
* indicate the share dividend
* hold elections for officers of the company.

Annual returns

The company annual return must:

* give the name and registered address of the company
* have details of all shares and shareholders and changes over the past year
* list the directors and the secretary
* detail any debts that the company may have.

The signed annual return must be sent with a fee to the Registrar within two weeks of the AGM. It is possible that your pharmacy company return will hardly differ from year to year.

Tax and VAT

This is best left to the accountant, but basically corporation tax must be paid on the profits from the accounting period and not later than nine months after that period. Customs and Excise deal with VAT and your pharmacy, unlike dispensing practices, must be registered for VAT.

So that is company law in a nutshell. As a future company director you will be expected to understand and abide by these laws as all others. Unfortunately, there is a great deal more to it than shown above. After all, thousands of solicitors and barristers have devoted their whole careers and made huge fortunes out of company law. Do not add to their fortunes unnecessarily by being unfamiliar with this complicated subject.

Forming your company

Now it's time to get on with forming the company, which will apply to, or notify, the PCO about its intention to dispense to NHS patients.

The first stage, of course, is to decide who will be the board members and major shareholders. In short, who is going into partnership to form your pharmacy company. That, of course, is your choice.

There are a number of considerations. The first instinct would be to have a normal practice meeting of the general practice partners and agree that you all should be directors of the board. That seems eminently reasonable, straightforward and sensible but, and there is a big but, what will happen should the partnership break up because a partner retires, moves or dies?

It could be that by that time the pharmacy will be quite a large, financially profitable company. Any departing partner or his estate will also have equity in the GP practice. The payment of both sums to the departing partner or his estate could be quite a problem for the remaining partners in both businesses.

It could be an even greater problem for a doctor coming into the medical partnership, who would probably be asked to buy a partnership share in addition to shares in the pharmacy at a very early stage in his career. In comparison the student loan would pale into insignificance.

I can offer no general solution to this but to take careful legal advice, bearing in mind the considerations mentioned above. The outcome is likely to be that all partners will be given a free choice, but that only those partners, as future directors, will have any influence on the business of the pharmacy.

A point to understand – it is not essential to have a pharmacist at this stage, so the question of him being a partner will not arise. Any 'body corporate' can apply to the NHS for a contract to provide pharmaceutical services and such 'bodies' are not required to have a pharmacist among their number.

The company name

As mentioned above, there are strict rules and regulations about a company name, so it must be considered with great care, but even then you may be asked to think again. The company name must not:

• be already registered or very similar to a registered name
• imply any connection with any government or local authority body
• be offensive
• be misleading to the public.

It is also advisable for it not to bear any close resemblance to the name of the medical practice. 'The Riverside Medical Practice' partners may well come to own an in-house pharmacy, but it would be better were it not called 'Riverside Pharmacy' or even carry the name of one or more of the doctors, otherwise patients and others may be unduly influenced one way or the other.

The preliminary meeting prior to the formal application to Companies House could be quite enjoyable as a name-choosing session.

The worst that can happen is that the Registrar will temporarily refuse your application until another name for the company is chosen. Have a few alternatives in mind.

Next you should apply to Companies House for Forms 10 and 12. This may be done by telephone (0870 333 3636). At the same time you should ask for their advice pack and even request a check on your proposed company name. Form 12 has to be sworn in the presence of a solicitor. This may or may not be expensive.

The formalities and essential documents

The essential formal documents that are required by Companies House are:

- the Memorandum of Association
- the Articles of Association

and statements carrying:

- details of the directors and the company secretary
- details of the shares to be issued when the company is incorporated
- details of compliance with the Companies Act.

The Memorandum of Association
This important document carries:

- the company name
- the location of the registered office
- details about the business of the company – in this case, a pharmaceutical retail and dispensing business
- general details about the company, including selling its shares, leasing equipment, etc
- details of the amount of the company share capital and the value and type of the shares, general, preferred or debenture
- a statement of the limited liability of the shareholders
- a clause stating that two or more shareholders wish to form the company and how many shares they will each hold.

The purpose of the Memorandum is to state the powers of the company and how it relates to the world in general.

The Articles of Association
The Articles determine the internal running of the company and its relationship with the shareholders. There should also be clauses covering the interrelationship of the shareholders.

The Articles should contain:

- a list of the types of shares together with the rights attached to each kind (this has been described earlier in the chapter)
- details of any restrictions on the issue of future shares
- any matters relating to the transfer of company shares
- the details of company officers, directors and secretary
- details of the payment to each officer
- information relating to the powers of the officers. These will include the right to deal in company property and to limit any debt the directors may run into in the company name.

Enclosed with the Articles will be a form which should be used to open a company bank account.

The next stage, having completed all the paperwork, is to send it with the fee, currently £20, to Companies House where it will be scrutinised. After a short period of time a Certificate of Incorporation will be sent, together with a company number.

Two financial steps must then be taken.

1   You should use the form that arrived with the Articles to open the company bank account.
2   You should then register for VAT with Customs and Excise.

At the same time as notifying you of the successful setting up of your pharmacy company, Companies House will inform the Inland Revenue, who will send the company a corporation tax return.

Every year, on the date the company was set up, the company must complete accounts which must be submitted to Companies House. The annual fee for this is presently £15.

It is permissible and sensible to change this account's reference date to 31 March, so that it corresponds with the corporation tax year. This may be done on Form 225, which can be downloaded from the Companies House website: www. companieshouse.gov.uk.

Profits

Profits are distributed to shareholders and the partners, as dividends. A voucher must accompany dividend payments and could be on company notepaper and should list:

- the date
- the number of shares
- the dividend paid
- the tax credit.

Tax

The dividend paid to shareholders by a limited company carries a tax credit. For the time being this is 10%. This means that a dividend of £540 is worth 90% of the total taxable value and the tax credit is one-ninth of £540, that is £60.

Finally

Even though your company has been accepted by Companies House, there is a final, extremely essential step and that is to register the pharmacy with the Royal Pharmaceutical Society of Great Britain. Without this registration it is prohibited in the strongest possible terms to trade as a 'chemist', whether in the NHS or not.

Chapter 6

The NHS application

Things are going well. You are now pretty well conversant with most of the law relating to pharmacy and business practice, and Companies House has registered the business. Even the taxman has been informed to await his share of your profits. The next stage is to get your pharmacy on the NHS list of pharmacies.

A very useful step first, however, would be to seek the support of the users of the health centre – the patients. How would they feel about not having to make a separate visit to the high street to have their prescriptions filled? Would it be a hardship or would they welcome the close proximity and cooperation of the pharmacist and the doctors with all the safety features involved in that cooperation?

Carrying out a survey such as that would, of course, let the cat out of the bag and warn the high-street pharmacist, so only do it when you are prepared to go ahead.

On the other hand, imagine how much having solid patient support would strengthen your case with the authority, whether it is an 'OFT application/notification' or a standard application under current regulations.

It is at this stage that it will be essential to employ a solicitor experienced in pharmacy applications, especially for a formal application. Before calling the solicitor in you should be sure that you have collected together all the paperwork needed to progress your application. The earlier chapters have given a pretty clear indication of what will be needed. If the solicitor has to do the legwork then you will be charged handsomely for it.

If the government follows through its intentions there will be two routes:

1   notification after deregulation has been formalised
2   formal application through the current procedure if 1 does not apply.

Notification

There are good reasons to believe that such a formal application will not be needed in many cases when the government gets around to implementing its own recommendations. Those recommendations were that there should be deregulation of the pharmacy entry rules in three cases:

1   retail developments of more than 15 000 square metres
2   pharmacies open for more than 100 hours a week
3   one-stop healthcare centres.

Regulation would remain for high-street pharmacies.

The effect of the changes will be a rapid growth in supermarket pharmacies, both in and out of town. After all, that was what the OFT was originally asked to consider. Whether the term 'retail developments of more than 15 000 square metres' will include new shopping malls rather than simply one large supermarket store is still a debatable point. No doubt one or more of the retail pharmacy chains will see to it through the courts that that is decided, sooner rather than later. If so, then the multiples will march in.

My own interpretation is that it is intended that any pharmacy will be permitted to provide NHS dispensing services in any shopping mall larger than 15 000 square metres without regulation. However, I do believe that pharmacy will object to this and that government may give way over this point in order to win their flagship *NHS Plan*[1] promise over one-stop health centres.

There will be few pharmacies that remain open more than 100 hours a week. To save having to do the maths, that comes to 16 hours a day, six days a week or $14\frac{1}{2}$ hours every day for a seven-day week. Of the ones that do open these hours the vast majority are going to be in larger towns, conurbations or transport termini where there is an almost constant demand for urgent medicines or a large population of addicts. Few doctors will be able to or want to use that exception to establish their own pharmacy.

The many medical practices that could well benefit from the OFT changes will be the ones with large premises or those prepared and able to extend their premises to include all the services needed under the definition 'a one-stop healthcare' centre.

The services mentioned in *The NHS Plan* include an optician, a dentist, a health visitor, a social worker and, the current topic, a pharmacy. *The NHS Plan* makes no stipulation that any of the services should be permanent services – not even the pharmacy, although it is common sense that that should be. The others could well be part-time.

That being so, the practice may consider entering into conversation with these other professionals with a view to them extending their practice by renting a consultation room within the newly extended, or existing premises. After all, they would benefit from the convenience of in-house referrals from the medical practice.

It has to be said, however, that in the current climate it may well be very difficult to attract any dentist into providing treatment under the NHS, even in a one-stop healthcare centre. If that is the only obstacle to fulfilling *The NHS Plan* criteria then the PCO may well be very understanding. If, however, you do manage to find a willing dentist, that must count greatly in your favour.

Consider the additional presence of the other professionals to be the loss leaders needed to be allowed to open a very profitable pharmacy business. The viability of the pharmacy was discussed in Chapter 2. Did you get the impression that it would be quickly going bankrupt?

Would you need or want financial help with the development of your premises? Then return to Chapter 1 where mention is made of NHS subsidies. If these are not available then such is the state of the economy today that it should be fairly simple to raise a loan under good terms from the usual commercial sources.

Yes, I hear you say, this is all very well, but is the government likely to make these changes that seem so appealing to medical practice and so abhorrent to pharmacy? Remember what pharmacy solicitor Mr David Reissner told *Pharmacy*

Magazine[2] readers in January 2004: 'The government's proposals may accelerate the ownership of pharmacies by GPs – an undesirable development'.

Mr Reissner is a well-respected lawyer from an impressive firm of London solicitors, who specialises in matters relating to pharmacy and he appears to agree with the author that change is in the air. Quite why he believes GP ownership to be an 'undesirable development' is hard to understand. After all, every GP-owned pharmacy will, by law, require a superintendent pharmacist to manage it. That being so, does it matter whether the company is owned by a chimney sweep, a health visitor or even a group of unemployed traffic wardens, just so long as the pharmacy is efficiently and legally run, according to the laws and regulations of the land and the code of ethics of the Pharmaceutical Society?

To say otherwise is to demean oneself and raise matters of professional jealousy. Indeed, there is good reason to believe that a GP-owned pharmacy in GP premises could well be better run than even a high-street pharmacy. GPs are, after all in the business of medicines and caring for their patients, the very patients who are most likely to obtain their medicines from that pharmacy. Any sub-standard practice or poor service will quite reasonably reflect back on the doctors themselves.

Indeed, even the NPA now agrees with this and has recently changed its rules to permit doctor-owned pharmacies to become members of that Association.

The government understands this and I believe that within a relatively short period of time this government will introduce the modifications they themselves made to the original OFT report of a year or so ago. They are certainly showing no inclination not to do so.

In any case, pharmacists as individual professionals, need not be concerned. Many more salaried posts could well become available and what is the difference between being employed by a large chain of pharmacies or a medical practice? Indeed, the salary and conditions for the pharmacist may be much better in a health centre. After all, the pharmacist will be seen to be an important member of the team due to proximity to the medical practice.

So, doctors, it would be as well to be prepared and not to miss the opportunity that may well be presented. Even if it is not presented in the way I suspect it will be, then you will at least have prepared the ground for an application through the current regulations. More of that later.*

The possible OFT application process

It is more than likely that the NHS will develop an official form for such applications with space for:

- applicant details
  - name and registered address of applicant pharmacy company
- health centre information
  - name and address of health centre where the pharmacy will be situated
  - evidence of presence in health centre of other professionals:

  (i)   optician: statement, signed, dated containing details of practice
  (ii)   dentist: statement, signed, dated with similar details

---

*****Latest developments**: In late August 2004 the government implied that even 'de-regulated' pharmacy applications may have to satisfy the 'necessary or desirable' clause but the opportunities for GPs remain.

    (iii)   health visitor: statement, signed, dated with similar details
    (iv)   others: statements, signed as before.

- evidence from health centre
  - statement of medical practice of willingness to become a one-stop primary care centre
  - evidence from the owners of the health centre of adequate premises for pharmacy as approved by the RPSGB.

- pharmacy information
  - statement of the pharmacy company as to their fitness to practise in the health centre
  - Pharmacy Registration Certificate from the Pharmaceutical Society
  - services to be provided by pharmacy company from the health centre
  - date of proposed commencement of service
  - name, address and registration number of superintendent pharmacist.

- signature of board member(s) of applicant company, senior GP partner and/or owners of the premises
- date.

It is unlikely that any PCO is going to just say 'Yes, OK' to a quick telephone call. Some formal application as the above may well be instituted by each PCO. It eliminates the current formal application procedure (see below), but still allows the PCO to examine the suitability of each application to determine whether the standards are suitable in every way.

    It seems reasonable that a notification could be refused on quality, premises or definition grounds, subject to appeal. Under the proposed changes it would not be reasonable or permissable for the notification to be refused simply because there is another pharmacy in the high street, for instance or because the company is owned by doctors. As an eminent past-chairman of the BMA Council used to emphasise: 'Words mean what words say' (Dr John Marks). In this case, deregulation means deregulation even in this limited fashion.

Formal application, the current procedure

From this stage onwards it is essential to have the expert advice of a solicitor experienced in pharmacy matters, especially in the application process. The fact that you have all the paperwork to hand and a working knowledge of the law and the regulations will be of help.

    The most important document you will need is: *The NHS (Pharmaceutical Services) Regulations 1992, No. 662*. The current version will incorporate all the amendments enacted since 1992 and there have been many.

    The Regulations set out who may apply for an NHS Pharmacy contract:

        application for inclusion in the pharmaceutical list may be made by registered pharmacists and persons lawfully conducting a retail pharmacy business in accordance with Section 69 of the Medicines Act 1968. These persons include registered pharmacists, partnerships of pharmacists and bodies corporate.

This is emphasised by *The Guidance on Procedures HSG(92)13*, which demands that all applications for inclusion in the pharmaceutical list must be rejected if they are not from pharmacists, partnerships of pharmacists or corporate bodies. At this stage, therefore, as the company is 'a body corporate' a pharmacist is not required.

There is another significant section:

> (2)   A person, other than a doctor or dentist –
>
>> (a)   who wishes to be included in a pharmaceutical list for the provision of pharmaceutical services from premises in a Health Authority's (HA) area or
>> (b)   who is already included in a pharmaceutical list but wishes –
>>
>>> (i)   to open, within an HA's area additional premises from which to provide the same or different pharmaceutical services
>>> (ii)   to change the premises from which he provides pharmaceutical services to other premises within that area from which he wishes to provide the same or different pharmaceutical services, or
>>> (iii) to provide from his existing premises in that area pharmaceutical services other than those already listed in relation to him,
>
> shall apply to the HA in the form set out in Part I of Schedule 3, and in this regulation 'applicant' and 'application shall be construed accordingly'

The clause specifying 'other than a doctor or dentist' is the precise reason why GPs should set up a separate company and why it is that the company applies, as a separate entity, rather than the doctors.

It may be of some interest that this:

(i)   gives an indication of the infamous loophole in the regulations, which has been the downfall of so many medical practices
(ii)   covers the relocation of premises.

Putting it concisely, there are six main classes of applications – those:

1   for a new contract in a town
2   for additional premises
3   for a change of premises, not a minor relocation
4   for the provision of additional services
5   for a change of premises which is a 'minor relocation'
6   for a change of ownership.

To these should be added:

7   an application within a rural area.

Of the above classes of applications, (1) to (4):

> (4)   ... shall be granted by the HA *only if it is satisfied that it is necessary or desirable to grant the application* in order to secure, in the neighbourhood in which the premises from which the applicant intends to provide the services are located, the adequate provision, by persons on the list, of the services, or some of the services, specified in the application.

Of 1 to 4 only 1 may be of direct interest to medical practices, although the others may have some attraction as alternative strategies.

Briefly, what clause (4) means is that if there is a chemist close by your premises the authority may reject your application unless the application shows persuasive reasons for it being accepted.

The most persuasive reason of all is that the pharmaceutical services you offer will take place within the health centre and that they will outdo the services provided in the high street. That is a factor that this government believes to be of great importance as a matter of convenience to patients, especially if the existing high-street pharmacy is some distance away. In that case, it may be *desirable* even if not *necessary*. Note that the clause says *'necessary or desirable'*, not *'and desirable'*. This is a point which can be exploited by your solicitor.

So, it may very well be worthwhile putting in an application under the Regulations (2)(a) above. Whereas, if there is a pharmacy within 100 yards or so, for instance, it would likely be a waste of time to do so. Such an application would fail under the *'necessary or desirable'* clause.

Applications of classes 2 to 6 may have some attraction as alternative strategies to practices who may be unable to set up their own pharmacy. There are sure to be many pharmacists who, on finding out that the practice has space to spare, may wish to take advantage of that space to improve the service and profitability of their own pharmacy. This may be under the 'minor location' clause.

There is no definition of a minor relocation, but it has been taken to mean that such a move would not significantly affect the services provided. Presumably, that means there would be no adverse effect on services as I cannot believe that any authority would refuse a move that had the effect of improving services.

That being the case, if a pharmacy does approach the practice with a relocation in mind then it is for the practice to do its sums properly, to act business-like and to get the best deal it can.

Remember, if the premises are owned by the practice then it is in a very strong position because, as any pharmacist will realise, an in-house pharmacy will catch virtually all the NHS dispensing. The position is so strong that the pharmacist may be content to take the practice or its pharmacy company into partnership if that is the only way of getting a foothold in the premises.

On the other hand, the practice may be in a position to buy out one of the high-street chemists and relocate that pharmacy into the health centre. That may seem an extreme step to take but, thinking of the profits involved, it may well be worth considering carefully.

The most likely effect is that a Dutch auction will follow, especially if the chains of pharmacies, as noted in Chapter 2, become involved. Don't omit to involve them if it will be profitable to do so and it usually will be.

Rural applications

Class 7 applications in rural areas are very special, mainly being of concern to dispensing doctors who fear the ingress of a pharmacy through the Clothier Regulations or the 'loophole'.

Any practice considering opening a pharmacy in a rural area must, and it cannot be emphasised too much, must, out of common courtesy, consult other dispensing practices that may have patients within the one-mile rule area.

If an application is successful then all those practices will lose dispensing rights for their patients within a one-mile radius of the new pharmacy. They may be less than amused – and it has happened.

Rural applications are made through the Clothier Regulations[3], which were set up, as mentioned in Chapter 1, to police the professional dispensing boundaries in these areas between dispensing doctors and pharmacists.

Any application by a pharmacy to dispense in a rural area is inevitably going to be vigorously opposed unless, of course, the application is a defensive one by the threatened practice of dispensing doctors themselves or, more precisely, their independent company.

These applications will have the advantage over any other pharmacy application of being early and of already having the ownership of suitable premises from which dispensing is being carried out.

Another advantage to the dispensing practice is that if a pharmacy application is refused, even its own, then another application may not be made for five years unless there have been 'substantial changes' to the area. This means a large population growth, for example.

Applications for pharmacies in rural areas must pass through three main hurdles:

1   rurality
2   the 'prejudice' clause
3   the 'necessary or desirable' clause.

Rurality

Important in Clothier applications is the fact of 'rurality', whether the area in question is truly rural. Although there is no quoted definition of rurality, such factors as population density and the provision of other local services such as shops, transport, schools will affect the decision.

Prejudice, the proper provision . . .

In the case of a rural, Clothier or Regulation 12, application the 'prejudice clause' includes 'prejudice to the proper provision of general medical or general pharmaceutical services to the area'. This provides a difficult defence for the medical practice because, by regulation, they do not provide pharmaceutical services. However, it may be possible for the doctors to prove that the pharmacist would not be able to comply fully with their terms of service because of the lack of funds from the small rural pharmacy. The pharmacist cannot, at this stage, depend on the assumption that an ESPS would be provided.

The medical practice may be able to argue that the sudden and drastic loss of their dispensing income would threaten the medical services provided by the practice. However, this is not the place to discuss that theme. It is better covered in *The Complete Dispenser*.[4]

Necessary or desirable

If the authority believes there to be no prejudice to either then it goes on to consider the 'necessary or desirable' clause. Once rurality has been disproven then the authority will almost inevitably decide that a pharmacy will be both necessary and desirable.

The loophole (q.v.)

The loophole in Regulation 12 has already been described (Chapter 1) and this may be helpful in its own right for pharmacy applications.

Closure of the loophole, as proposed by the DDA Ltd, GPC and pharmacy, may, just may, prevent pharmacy applications, while at the same time as ring-fencing current dispensing practices to protect pharmacies in so-called market towns. This ring-fencing is just likely to make the total destruction of dispensing by doctors a greater possibility in the future, that is, if regulation changes mooted earlier by the Fifth Health Committee report don't get there first.

On the other hand, the author's understanding of the proposed DDA Ltd changes is that the protection of the rural dispensing practice will be less robust than the protection of the market town pharmacy. This will mean that the larger rural practices will still have to keep an even more wary eye open than usual for a pharmacy takeover bid, in which case, the next several pages will be helpful.

The Pharmacy Application Form

The application to the authority must be made on the proper form, known as Schedule 3, Part 1 or a copy of it.

There are two classes of application:

1 full
2 preliminary consent.

An application for preliminary consent allows the applicant not to state the address of his premises. Indeed, at the time of application he may not have any. However, a successful application will be valid only for 12 months, extendable for another 12 months by the authority if sufficient notice is given. The full application, if any, must be made during that period and, if made, must be granted, but only if an address of the proposed premises is given to the authority.

The strictures for an application for preliminary consent are identical to those for a full application. All it does is to allow the chemist to find out whether a pharmacy would be allowed without, at the time of application, going to the trouble and expense of buying premises.

Northamptonshire Heartlands **NHS**
Primary Care Trust

PRIMARY CARE PRACTITIONER SERVICES

SCHEDULE 3, PART 1

APPLICATION FOR INCLUSION IN A PHARMACEUTICAL LIST OR INCLUSION IN A LIST IN RESPECT OF DIFFERENT SERVICES OR PREMISES*

To the Northamptonshire Heartlands Primary Care Trust

1   I/we...

of...

(a)   apply in my/our own right/on behalf of .... to be included in the merged Health Authority's Pharmaceutical List for the provision of services listed in paragraph 6 below. I/we are not already included in any pharmaceutical list kept by the Health Authority,

(b)   am/are already included in a Pharmaceutical List kept by the merged Health Authority, but apply to open additional premises for the provision of the services listed in paragraph 6 below,

(c)   am/are already included in a Pharmaceutical List kept by the merged Health Authority, but apply to relocate the premises from which I/we are to provide the services listed in paragraph 6 below;

(d)   am/are already included in a Pharmaceutical List kept by the Authority, but apply to provide from my/our existing premises additional services to those already provided;

(e)   am/are already included in a Pharmaceutical List kept by the merged Health Authority, but apply to withdraw the provision of a service/services from an existing premises.

2.   *(To be completed only by persons applying under paragraph 1(a), (b), (c) or 4)*

(a)   The premises from which I/we wish to provide those services are at

....

....

(b)   Those premises are:
☐   already constructed
☐   already in my/our possession/not yet in my/our possession (be rental, leasehold or freehold)
☐   under negotiation
☐   registered by the Royal Pharmaceutical Society of Great Britain
If so, state reference number...

3.   *(To be completed only by persons who are included in a Pharmaceutical List kept by the Authority)* The premises from which I/we provide pharmaceutical services are at
....
....

The services I/we provide from those premises are ....
....
....

4.   (To be completed only by persons applying under paragraph 1(a) who are proposing to provide services at premises from which services are already provided i.e. change of ownership)

The name of the chemist who is providing services from the premises named in paragraph 2(a) above is ....

The provision of services from those premises will be continuous/interrupted by *(state period)*...

5. *(To be completed only by persons applying under paragraph 1(c) above)*
The relocation is for the following reasons:-

....

....

....

(To be completed only is the applicant considers relocation to be minor)
I/We consider the relocation to be minor for the following reasons:-

....

....

The provision of services by me/us will be continuous/interrupted by *(state period)*

....

6. *(To be completed by all applicants)*
I/We propose to provide/withdraw the following pharmaceutical services
- ☐ PROVISION OF DRUGS
- ☐ Provision of the following listed appliances:-
- ☐ OXYGEN CYLINDERS
- ☐ STOMA APPLIANCES
- ☐ ELASTIC HOSIERY
- ☐ TRUSSES
- ☐ OTHER APPLIANCES (please specify)
....
- ☐ OTHER SERVICES (please specify)
....

7. *(To be completed by all applicants except those proposing either to provide services from premises from which the services listed in paragraph 6 are already provided or to change within the neighbourhood the premises from which pharmaceutical services listed in paragraph 6 are already provided)*

In my/our view the provision of the proposed services are the premises named in this application is necessary or desirable in order to secure in the neighbourhood in which the premises are located the adequate provision of those services by persons in the list of services for the following reasons:-

....

....

8. I/We undertake that if my/our application is granted, I/we will provide/continue to provide the pharmaceutical services specified in paragraph 6 at the premises specified in paragraph 2.

Signed ....

Date ....

*The sections or words which do not apply should be deleted as necessary.

Please send completed form to Primary Care Practitioner Services, Northamptonshire Heartlands PCT, Lancaster House, Isebrook Hospital, Irthlingborough Road, Wellingborough, Northants, NN8 1LP

h:\practitioner services\pharmacy\forms\reg4(2).doc

With thanks to the Northamptonshire Heartlands Primary Care Trust.

The doctors' pharmacy company could apply for preliminary consent before making any changes to the original health centre premises.

1   *Question 1.* The name and address of the applicant should be completed here and the inappropriate sections (a) to (e) deleted. They list the alternative kinds of application.
2   *Question 2.* This allows space for the address from which services are intended to be provided. If the application is a preliminary one then this could be completed with the words 'Preliminary Application'. There are also alternative descriptions of the premises, some of which should be deleted.
3   *Question 3.* This allows space for the address of persons already on the HA pharmaceutical list and for the services provided from that address. Their application will be easier for the reasons mentioned above.
4   *Question 4.* This seeks details of a change of ownership, if any.
5   *Question 5.* This asks for the reasons for the relocation, why it is said to be 'minor' and for how long pharmaceutical services will be interrupted during the relocation process.
6   *Question 6.* This consists of a list of pharmaceutical services, which may or may not be provided by the applicant. There are tick-boxes. The more boxes ticked, the more likely the application is to succeed.
7   *Question 7.* Very little space is provided for the completion of this question despite its importance. It asks applicants to state why they believe the services they intend to provide from their premises are 'necessary or desirable'.

Careful thought should be given to this one as it could well be the make or break question. Remember *The NHS Plan* and the government's wish for patient convenience and one-stop centres. Quote the relevant sections from it. They are to be found in Chapter 1 of this book.

8   *Question 8.* The final question seeks the applicant's signature in confirmation that he will do as he says and provide the listed services from the listed premises.

The completed form must then be sent to the appropriate primary care practitioner services of the appropriate PCT.

Strictures upon the authority

They may grant the application for some or all of the services specified in it. Before or on granting the application they must:

- notify certain bodies – see below
- consider any other providers of pharmaceutical services and other matters
- notify certain groups – as below
- notify the applicant about the appeals procedure.

Consider Section 12 on rural applications separately and specially. Inform the applicant of how much time will be granted to him before services must commence.

Notification

On receipt of the application the authority must, 'as soon as is practicable', notify:

- the Local Medical Committee (LMC)
- the Local Pharmaceutical Committee (LPC)
- any person on the pharmaceutical list who may be affected
- any other HA whose area is within 2 km of the premises
- any future equivalent to the Community Health Council (CHC).

These bodies have 30 days to send their observations on the application to the authority.

Determination of the application

The authority must consider everything carefully and this includes:

- the effect on pharmaceutical services already being provided
- any other relevant information
- any comments from the groups notified above.

It may or may not decide to hold an oral hearing, but if it does decide to, then involved persons will be given not less than 14 days' notice. None of the affected may be represented by any counsel or solicitor at this preliminary oral hearing.

No provider of general medical or pharmaceutical services may take part in the decision-making process, but the LPC and the LMC may do so.

Two or more applications may be considered at the same time. If one has premises and the other does not then it is probable that the one with premises will be considered first, as suggested in the solicitor's advice earlier in this book. The one that owns premises is very likely to be the medical practice – so get prepared early.

Notification of the decision

The authority must notify the same groups of its decision as it notified of the application. It must include with the notice a statement of the reasons for the decision and the rights of appeal.

Appeals

An appeal on the authority's decision may be made to the Secretary of State by:

- the applicant
- any person given notice of the application (as above)
- any other affected authority.

The appeal must be made within 30 days from the date the decision was notified. If there is more than one appeal in the case of multiple applications, then they will all be considered together.

The Secretary of State may dismiss an appeal that has no reasonable grounds or is frivolous. On the other hand he may call an oral hearing to be held by one or more persons he appoints for that purpose.

Affected persons will have not less than 14 days' notice and they and the appellant may, this time, have counsel or a solicitor to either speak for them or to advise them.

The Secretary of State will give notice of his decision as soon as is practicable to all the same bodies as before.

There is no further right of appeal although some may consider a Judicial Review to be warranted after taking detailed and thorough legal advice. Judicial Reviews consider whether the proper legal steps have been taken by the authority, the appeal body or by the Secretary of State. If there has been any inadvertent misuse or mistake of the legal process then the case may be reopened, reconsidered or, even determined by the court.

The Northern Ireland application form

The Northern Ireland application form is known as: HS28 (revised 10/97) AI, Part I, Regulation 6(2) Form A.[5]

It is a little less clear than the English form and takes up three pages instead of two. The information requested includes the applicant's name, address and the address of the proposed premises. The authority also asks whether the premises are already constructed and in the possession of the applicant. Evidence of ownership in the form of a title or lease, together with a detailed map of location must be submitted with the form. Following this request are questions relating to the services to be provided and the name of the registered pharmacist who will be in charge. Finally, a 'necessary or desirable' clause awaits a signature from the applicant.

It appears that there is no intermediate step of preliminary consent as there is in England.

The completed form is sent to the appropriate Health and Social Services Board.

The remaining procedure broadly follows that of the English system 'across the water'. However, there is great prejudice against dispensing by doctors in Northern Ireland, so a pharmacy application in a doctor-dispensing area would seem to be more likely to be met with approval.

Assuming your application has been approved by the authority, the next stage is to prepare and staff the new pharmacy.

References

1 Department of Health (2000) *The NHS Plan*. Stationery Office, London.
2 Reissner D (2004) Talking Point. *Pharmacy Magazine*. **January**: 6.
3 *NHS (General Medical & Pharmaceutical Services) Amendment Regulations, 1983, No. 313 (The original 'Clothier' Regulations)*. Stationery Office, London.
4 Roberts D (2002) *The Complete Dispenser*. Communications International Group, London.
5 *HS28 (revised 10/97) AI, Part I, Regulation 6(2) Form A*. Stationery Office, London.

Chapter 7

Staffing the pharmacy

It should go without saying that the most important member of your staff will be the superintendent pharmacist. Your pharmacy cannot legally function as a pharmacy, either in or out of the NHS, without this member of staff.

You may consider it good policy to invite him to become involved in the design stage of the pharmacy, not only because his Code of Ethics, as described below, entreats him to work in premises of a 'professional character', but also because it would be a shrewd political move. A pharmacist who has been trusted sufficiently to be involved in planning the pharmacy in which he works is likely to have increased loyalty to that business. It will be 'his' business.

The next several pages describe the duties, and the Terms of Service of pharmacists together with the Code of Ethics of the Pharmaceutical Society. All this is in order that the interview panel will be better informed and will, hopefully, choose the right candidates and, eventually, the right superintendent pharmacist to carry the project through to completion. A lot depends on that.

The pharmacist

The pharmacist will be discussed under seven headings:

1   the definition of a pharmacist
2   professional organisations
3   the code of ethics
4   the terms of service
5   negligence
6   confidentiality
7   a contract of employment.

What is a pharmacist?

It was not until the Pharmacy Act of 1852 that the Pharmaceutical Society was given powers to examine potential pharmacists and to prohibit anyone from practising the profession of pharmacy without a certificate from the Society. Before that time apothecaries, chemists and druggists dispensed the mostly poorly effective medicines.

The Pharmacy Act of 1954, 100 years later, confirmed and governed the education and organisation of the profession.

In 1988 the Pharmaceutical Society was granted the right in future to be known as the Royal Pharmaceutical Society of Great Britain (RPSGB). Its members are defined as registered pharmaceutical chemists and only registered members may buy and sell drugs or dispense medicines. Their names and addresses are kept on a register[1] by the Registrar of the Society if he is satisfied that they have qualified by examination and have a certificate of competence to practise. The Register is updated annually.

The Society must issue a certificate of registration to qualified pharmacists and the pharmacist must prominently display it at his place of business. It is a criminal offence to display a forged certificate.

The interview panel should demand sight of the certificate of registration and verify its authenticity with the Society before considering employing any pharmacist.

There are three main branches of pharmacy:

1 community
2 hospital
3 the pharmaceutical industry.

There are 16 schools of pharmacy in the universities of this country, all of them with four-year undergraduate degree programmes recognised by the Pharmaceutical Society and all conferring the MPharm degree on successful candidates, hopefully with Hons.

The successful awarding of the MPharm is followed by a year of pre-registration training either in the community or a hospital pharmacy. At the end of this the pharmacist must pass the Pharmaceutical Society's registration examination and only then will the candidate's name be entered on the Annual Register of Pharmaceutical Chemists. He will then be permitted to practise as a pharmacist and will remain on the Register by payment of an annual fee unless his name is removed following an episode of malpractice or some other disciplinary offence.

Professional organisations

The RPSGB is the regulatory and standard-setting body for pharmacy. No pharmacist is permitted to practice unless their name is currently on its register, formally entitled *The Annual Register of Pharmaceutical Chemists*. Malpractice by the pharmacist may lead to the removal of their name in a similar fashion to that of the doctor who faces a General Medical Council (GMC) disciplinary enquiry.

In addition to regulating pharmacists the Society also regulates the premises of community chemists. Readers have already been advised to seek the advice of the RPSGB about their own premises, if in doubt.

The terms of reference of the Pharmaceutical Society are to:

- accredit undergraduate pharmacy courses
- promote the interests of pharmacy and pharmacists
- regulate the profession
- regulate pharmacy premises.

Until the Blair government introduced its Commission for the Regulation of Healthcare Professions (CRHP), now known, somewhat pompously, as the Council for Healthcare Regulatory Excellence (CHRE), the profession of pharmacy, like the medical profession through the GMC, was truly self-governing. However, health secretary Alan Milburn thought it wise not to trust the professions to govern themselves any longer, so he introduced CRHP as a super-regulatory body with the power to overrule any decision of the professional organisations.

In March 2004 the GMC found a doctor not guilty of the offence with which he had been charged, only to find that CRHP thought otherwise and demanded that the doctor be 'retried'. The result of the GMC appeal against this intrusion is still awaited. Pharmacists should be aware that self-regulation of the profession no longer exists.

In no way is the Pharmaceutical Society a trade organisation as, in parallel with the GMC, it takes no part in trade-union negotiations over the terms and service of the work of pharmacists. It is a professional body.

Again, rather like the GMC, the RPSGB is undergoing internal change at present and the pharmacy press is full of the constitutional wranglings between participants and members. The outcome of these is still unclear.

The Council of the Society currently consists of 21 elected members and three members appointed by the Privy Council.

Erring pharmacists may well find themselves facing The Statutory Committee of the RPSGB, which consists of five members from its Council plus a legally qualified chairman appointed by the Privy Council.

The Statutory Committee considers the cases of pharmacists whose probable misdeeds have been referred to it by others. Not only does the Committee consider the actions of the pharmacist, but also those of his employees. Information may not only be passed to the Committee by members of the public, the courts and the police, but also by its own team of inspectors who, sometimes incognito, visit pharmacies that are under suspicion.

In similar fashion to the GMC Screening Committee, the information received is scrutinised and a decision is made whether to go ahead with an enquiry.

No doubt these enquiries are as terrifying to pharmacists as GMC enquiries are to doctors. They may result either in a striking off the register, a reprimand or an exoneration. Subject to appeal, that used to be the end of the matter. However, the formation of CRHP has meant that the Commission or the Health Secretary may overrule the Society and demand a further hearing.

As we have seen, the Commission has already overruled one GMC 'not guilty' decision (March 2004).

Pharmacy organisations

Pharmaceutical Services Negotiating Committee (PSNC)
The Pharmaceutical Services Negotiating Committee (PSNC) is the group that negotiates the terms and conditions of service for pharmacists There are local branches – LPCs – throughout the country consisting of locally elected pharmacists. It has counterparts in the other countries of the UK and is a very effective organisation; some may say, in many ways more effective than the GPC.

Royal Pharmaceutical Society of Great Britain (RPSGB)
The RPSGB is the national regulatory body for pharmacy and it sets the standards for entry to the profession in a similar fashion to the GMC for doctors. No pharmacist may practice unless his name is listed on the Register of the Society.

In addition to that important function the Society promotes and maintains the ethical standards of pharmacy in this country.

Similar organisations exist in Northern Ireland (Pharmaceutical Society of Northern Ireland) and Scotland (Scottish Pharmaceutical General Council).

National Pharmaceutical Association (NPA)

The NPA was founded in 1921 as the national body of community pharmacy owners. Its aims are to promote, improve and protect community pharmacy. It currently has members in 11 000 community pharmacies in the UK.

It does not negotiate with government, but it does lobby very effectively. As will be seen later, not only does it educate and promote pharmacy and pharmacists, but it also maintains standards and it even helps design new pharmacies.

The NPA incorporates the Chemists Defence Association Ltd and a couple of insurance companies. There are branches of the NPA throughout the UK. It is based in St Albans, Hertfordshire.

Chemists Defence Association (CDA)

The CDA is a wholly owned subsidiary of the NPA. It provides professional indemnity cover of up to £10 million for professional errors by its members and, importantly, their employees and locums.

It will also provide defence, legal advice, representation and help on professional business matters. Its staff are well-versed in all the legal matters discussed earlier in this book (Chapter 4).

Pharmacy Mutual Insurance Company

A branch of the NPA, the PMIC provides pharmacists with general insurance needs at competitive prices. Full information may be obtained either through the company or through the NPA.

Pharmacists Defence Association

This organisation advertises that it provides robust legal support in dispute situations in primary care pharmacy. There is an on-line advice centre to support pharmacists. (www.the-pda.org)

Ulster Chemists Association (UCA)

The UCA is a benevolent society.

Proprietary Association of Great Britain

The PAGB is the trade association of the manufacturers of OTC medicines and food supplements. Its aim is to promote responsible consumer healthcare.

British Retail Consortium

The BRC is a trade association working on behalf of the retail industry, including pharmacy. It campaigns, informs and facilitates dialogue for retailers. It regularly publishes reports and guidelines on areas of the retail industry.

Institute of Pharmacy Management (IPM)

The aims of the Institute are 'to promote and inspire education, research and excellence in pharmacy management', and that does include community pharmacy. Members are encouraged to develop their skills by means of ongoing personal professional development.

Primary Care Pharmacists Association (PCPA)

The PCPA was recently founded to improve the quality of pharmacy services and make best uses of resources in primary care. Members are able to meet their peers for support and to foster further development. The association provides a series of local education events throughout the country and allows members to publish their own work.

Rural Pharmacists Association

This Association was recently wound up after achieving its main purpose following the agreement of pharmacy with the DDA Ltd and the GPC. The effect of the agreement was to limit the further expansion of dispensing by doctors.

Young Pharmacists Group (YPG)

The YPG is dedicated to promoting fresh ideas in pharmacy to ensure that the profession remains youthful in outlook. It claims to be at the cutting edge of pharmacy political debate and has promoted a number of international events.

The Scottish Pharmaceutical Federation

A similar organisation to the NPA, the SPF represents the owners of more than 1000 community pharmacies in Scotland – except Boots the Chemists.

Contact details for the above organisations are:

- British Retail Consortium, 5 Grafton Street, London, W1X 3LB
- Chemists Defence Association, 38–42 St Peter's Street, St Albans, Herts, AL1 3NP
- Institute of Pharmacy Management International, 14 Mamignot Close, Bearstead, Maidstone, Kent, ME14 4PT
- Pharmaceutical Society of Northern Ireland, 73 University Street, Belfast, BT7 1HL
- Pharmacy Mutual Insurance Co Ltd, 38 St Peter's Street, St Albans, Herts, AL1 3NP
- Scottish Pharmaceutical Federation, 135 Wellington Street, Glasgow, G2 2XD
- Scottish Pharmaceutical General Council, 42 Queen Street, Edinburgh, EH2 3NH
- Ulster Chemists Association, 73 University Street, Belfast, BT7 1HL
- Proprietary Association of Great Britain www.pagb.co.uk
- Primary Care Pharmacists Association www.pcpa.org.uk
- Young Pharmacists Group, PO Box 2641, Birmingham, B1 3EB.

The Code of Ethics of pharmacists[2]

The Code of Ethics of the Royal Pharmaceutical Society, and therefore of pharmacists, is, as would be hoped and expected, a very long document. It was adopted, after considerable consultation by the Council of the Society, as late as 1992 and is regarded as governing the conduct of all pharmacists both within and outside the practice of pharmacy. A breach could, according to the circumstances, form the basis of a complaint of misconduct.

There are nine *Principles*, each followed by relevant *Obligations*, which, in turn, are followed by appropriate *Guidance* on how to follow the obligations.

What follows here is, necessarily, but a brief description of the whole. It is well worthwhile asking the Pharmaceutical Society, even at this stage, for sight of a full copy. It is very revealing.

Principles and obligations

The nine principles that every pharmacist must observe are:

1   The pharmacist's prime concern must be for the patient and other members of the public

Following this there are no fewer than 24 obligations relating to patient trust, the purchase and sale of drugs or other items, a ban on tobacco sales, promotional campaigns, mail-order sales and many, many other topics.

Following the list of obligations there are several pages of *Guidance* on how to follow the obligations. For instance, every pharmacist must be competent in English to be able to do his job safely; he must not let his conscience interfere with his duties; he must keep up to date; not use counterfeit medicines and take care over drug misuse by patients. Again, there is much, much more.

It is this section that deals thoroughly with the provision of medicines.

2   A pharmacist must uphold the honour and dignity of the profession and ... not bring it into disrepute

This is straightforward, consisting of standards of behaviour and the use or misuse of qualifications. It also bans any pharmacist, even one who holds a doctorate, from using the title 'Doctor'.

3   A pharmacist must at all times have regard to the law and regulations applicable and maintain a high standard of professional conduct etc

Effectively this obliges the pharmacist to keep abreast of all laws and regulations at all times.

4   A pharmacist must respect the confidentiality of information acquired ... relating to a patient and a patient's family ...

The pharmacist must restrict the access of his staff to confidential information and make sure that those who do have access are aware of the principle of confidentiality. Computers must have password entry systems. There are no fewer than nine paragraphs of detailed guidance on this. A separate discussion on pharmacy confidentiality appears later in this chapter.

5   A pharmacist must keep abreast of pharmaceutical knowledge in order to maintain a high standard of professional competence ...

Continuing education is an uncontroversial principle. The pharmacist's responsibilities are set out in *Standards of Good Professional Practice*. These principles follow the line drawn in the case of *Crawford* v. *Board of Governors of Charing Cross Hospital (1953)*: 'once improvements become known, they may not be ignored ... specialists must keep abreast of developments in their field.'

There is here a warning for the pharmacist who takes on new roles or additional duties. By doing so he holds himself out as an expert and will be judged by a higher standard rather than with the average pharmacist.

6   A pharmacist must neither agree to practise under any conditions that compromise professional independence or judgement nor impose such conditions on other pharmacists

Here are to be found the duties of the superintendent pharmacist, which the GP-owned pharmacy will need to employ. It is worth quoting in full:

Employment as a superintendent pharmacist

6.3 By law a superintendent pharmacist is responsible for the management of the business so far as it concerns the keeping, preparing, dispensing and supplying of medicinal products.

6.4   In respect of all registered retail pharmacy premises owned by the business of which he is superintendent pharmacist, that pharmacist is professionally responsible for:

(a)   the observance of all legal and professional requirements
(b)   compliance with the professional standards currently accepted in pharmacy
(c)   the efficiency and quality of the pharmaceutical service provided by the business
(d)   the choice of suppliers of pharmaceutical goods and services to the business
(e)   in relation to the pharmaceutical service, the recruitment, management, training of staff and the allocation of duties to suitably competent staff
(f)   the conditions prevailing within each community pharmacy premises
(g)   the settlement of all questions concerning the nature and extent of the pharmaceutical service or which involve in any way pharmaceutical knowledge or professional conduct
(h)   ensuring that each employee pharmacist has sufficient knowledge of English language to enable that pharmacist to communicate effectively with all those to whom service are provided.

Guidance

The superintendent pharmacist may carry total responsibility if, as a result of his neglect or inactivity, a director is permitted to exercise functions which are the superintendent pharmacist's responsibility.

In short, the *Guidance* tells you, the directors, not to poke your nose into professional matters.

7   A pharmacist or a pharmacy owner should, in the public interest provide information about available professional services. Publicity must not claim or imply any superiority over the professional services provided by other pharmacists or pharmacies, must be dignified and must not bring the profession into disrepute.

Here in the *Guidance* is a definition of professional services and they include:

1   dispensing of prescriptions
2   the collection of prescriptions and delivery of dispensed medicines
3   maintenance of patient medication records
4   response to symptoms described in pharmacies (counter prescribing)
5   sale or supply of medicinal products
6   sale or supply of surgical dressings or appliances
7   sale or supply of poisons and chemicals
8   facilities for the sale or supply of hearing aids

9   diagnostic testing services, e.g. pregnancy testing, blood pressure testing or blood analysis
10   provision of pharmaceutical services to nursing homes, residential homes and sheltered housing
11   provision of health education and healthcare information
12   sale of goods, supply of services or the provision of advice where the pharmacist uses his scientific and pharmaceutical knowledge.

Among other strictures the *Obligations* tell the pharmacist that all publicity must be legal, decent and truthful. As an aside, some dispensing doctors will have had some doubts about this one during attempted applications by pharmacists to take over dispensing practices.

The *Guidance* adds that all forms of communication are embraced in it – leaflets, newspapers and even packaging. There will be one or two ex-dispensing practice GPs who will raise their eyebrows here, but possibly the *Guidance* only applies within the profession. Professional, practice leaflets and the information within them is covered here in some detail. This will be of use to your pharmacy, as will be the advice about advertising.

8   A pharmacist offering services directly to the public must do so in premises which reflect the professional character of the pharmacy

The obligation of the pharmacist is to ensure that inside and out the pharmacy within which he works meets the *Standards of Good Professional Practice*. In short, as the *Guidance* says, the appearance must be 'dignified and reflect the professional nature of the pharmacy'. The *Guidance* also determines how signs indicating the pharmacy should be designed and displayed. It even suggests that the approval of the Council of the Society should be obtained in some circumstances.

9   A pharmacist must at all times endeavour to cooperate with professional colleagues and members of other healthcare professions so that patients and public may benefit

The *Obligations* here emphasise exactly why the medical practice must set up its own, independent pharmacy company with no financial or other links with the general practice business. Under 'Association with medical practitioners' pharmacists are told:

1   not to enter into any association with doctors that may compromise their professional independence.

Does this mean that a superintendent pharmacist can never enter partnership with the doctors in the pharmacy enterprise? Must he always remain an employee? It rather looks that way.

2   to cooperate closely, professionally, with doctors but to:
   – ensure patients have freedom to ensure where their prescriptions are dispensed
   – ensure, wherever possible, that patients consent before their prescription is directed to a particular pharmacy.

These are the professional standards under which your pharmacist should work. Now for his Terms of Service under the NHS.

Terms of Service of an NHS pharmacy contractor

A number of official documents are included in the Terms of Service:

- the Regulations
- *The Drug Tariff*
- procedures of the NHS disciplinary committee
- procedures of the Tribunal Committee
- the procedures of the appeals committees of both the above.

It must be said here that the whole of the Terms of Service under which the pharmacist works are being renegotiated to develop a New Contract. Details of this are difficult to come by at the time of writing.

Under the *NHS (Pharmaceutical Services) Regulation 1992, Schedule 2*[3] all NHS pharmacists are contracted with the authority to:

- dispense NHS prescriptions promptly
- observe minimum opening hours. At the time of writing, the detail of this is currently being discussed as part of the pharmacists' New Contract.

The provision of pharmaceutical services

The provision of pharmaceutical services is covered under 14 headings and numerous subheadings. What follows is an extraction from this section.

1 A prescription presented at a pharmacy should be dispensed promptly or if that is not possible, within a reasonable time period.
2 Any drug or medicine provided must comply with the formula within *The British National Formulary*,[4] *The Drug Tariff*[5] or *The Pharmacopeia*[6] or other standard works.
3 Medicines must only be dispensed against a prescription form signed by a doctor or dentist.
4 The pharmacist may use his knowledge and experience to fill in gaps omitted by the prescriber, for instance, dosage and pack size.
5 The pharmacist may provide the minimum pack size for contraceptives, oral antibiotics and other named preparations.
6 There is a similar freedom for the chemist with hygroscopic preparations, liquids for addition to bath water and other named categories.
7 However, the chemist must follow the prescriber's instructions if it is the intention of the prescriber to provide less than the calendar pack.
8 Calendar packs and special containers are defined.
9 The pharmacist may dispense an urgent drug without a prescription if the prescriber is known to the pharmacist and requests him to do so and agrees to provide the form within 72 hours. This does not apply to scheduled drugs.
10 The pharmacist must only dispense scheduled drugs against a properly written prescription and with the other precautionary measures. The Shipman Enquiry report will inevitably tighten this up even further.

11   If a generic is prescribed the pharmacist may substitute an identical drug, but not a branded drug.

12   The above may apply to combination preparations only if the combination has a non-proprietary name.

13   Suitable containers must be used.

14   Pharmacists must not offer any inducement to anybody in any form for the giving of an order for medicines or drugs.

The New Contract may add another few clauses to the above, ones that allow pharmacists to prescribe certain drugs and another about repeat dispensing are very much on the cards.

There then follows a long section about premises and hours, but as these are under discussion in the New Contract negotiations it seems likely that the position will change shortly.

Provision of drugs and appliances

Drugs may only be dispensed under the direct supervision of a superintendent pharmacist. That sentence is quite categorical, but there are many members of the pharmacy profession who wish to loosen the bonds a little to allow them to undertake new roles and community tasks, such as visiting nursing homes, without having to cease dispensing medicines. The New Contract may have something to say about that.

All employed pharmacists must be on the Register and not suspended or erased from it. Their names must be given to the authority if requested.

The pharmacist must make arrangements for the measuring of patients for appliances where necessary.

Remuneration of chemists

All necessary records of supplemental services that have been carried out must be made available to the authority and entry to the premises must be given at all reasonable times for the authority to inspect that those services are being properly provided.

Payments will be made according to *The Drug Tariff.*

A suggestion for the pay scale for your own superintendent pharmacist was discussed in Chapter 2.

Charges

The pharmacist must observe the prescription charge regulations and must not charge for containers.

Professional standards

The pharmacist must maintain the standards as set out by the RPS. The pharmacist will also be responsible for ensuring that employed pharmacists obey those standards.

Complaints

The Terms of Service set out the complaints procedure in some detail and demand that a notice about this be prominently displayed on the premises. The final paragraph in this section demands that the pharmacist must cooperate with any investigation into his behaviour by the authority.

Supplemental services

The service mentioned here is the giving of advice for the safekeeping and correct administration of drugs to nursing homes. The advice need not be given by the pharmacist nor need he be the supplier of medicines to that home. There is no mention that the pharmacist should inform the GP either of his advice or even visit. There is mention that a record should be kept to allow payment to be made.

Additional professional services

These consist of:

- producing a practice leaflet which contains the pharmacist's professional qualifications and full details of his pharmacy
- displaying a statutory number of health promotion leaflets on his premises
- keeping patient medical records of patients exempt from charges or who may have difficulty understanding how to take their prescribed medicines.

Confidentiality

This is a major matter for any health professional and applies equally to those employed as to the principal himself. It should be included in any employee's contract of employment.

It has already been mentioned when describing the pharmacist's Code of Ethics, but it will do no harm to repeat the appropriate part of the Code here, in full:

> A pharmacist must respect the confidentiality of information acquired in the course of professional practice relating to patients and their families. Such information shall not be disclosed to anyone without the consent of the patient or appropriate guardian unless the interest of the public or the patient requires such a disclosure.

The Data Protection Act

All pharmacists and pharmacies must register under the Data Protection Act because they hold a considerable amount of information about patients. The rather confusing and unclear Data Protection Act governs how it should be kept and used.

Any interview panel should be aware that the Data Protection Act was amended fairly recently with the inclusion in it of a further right for job applicants. I wonder how many people know that candidates now have the right to examine any notes, written or otherwise, made during the interview.

No longer are you able to write such pithy aide-memoires as 'Fat, lazy slob, totally unsuitable' unless you are sure that those comments can be sustained in an employment tribunal if challenged by an applicant who felt they had been discriminated against.

It is important to become familiar with this Act although advice may need to be taken from a solicitor.

The pharmacist should consider the kind of data that will be gathered and must be sure that the registry with the Data Protection Act covers it. If not, then the registry should be updated so that it does.

There should be one person within the pharmacy whose duty it is to ensure that the business is registered under the Act and that these updates are regularly made.

Still on the subject of confidentiality, every NHS organisation employs a Caldicott Guardian – a healthcare professional responsible for safeguarding confidential patient information.

Before disclosing patient information the Caldicott Principles should be followed.

1 Justify the purpose.
2 Do not use identifiable information unless it is necessary.
3 Use the minimum amount of such information.
4 Access to such information should be on a 'need to know' basis.
5 Everyone in the pharmacy must be aware of their responsibilities.

Pharmacies should have standard operating procedures to ensure that all employees, including locum pharmacists, are fully aware of all this.

All confidential information must be effectively and safely secured. Hard copies must be locked away and computer copies must be protected by a password and, possibly, a firewall.

No identifiable patient information should be disclosed to anyone without the express and written consent of the patient involved. This brings us into direct conflict with the present Secretary of State for Health who is hell-bent on gaining identifiable information without the need to seek the permission of the patient. The conflict needs to be resolved, but until then my position is that the politician should be ignored and the patient's rights upheld. They must be paramount at all times.

Further and current information on confidentiality should be obtained from the PSNC, the NPA or the RPS.

Access to Health Records Act

Any patient or a person acting on his behalf can ask for access to non-computerised medical records about post-November 1991 information. The records involved will include patient medication records. The pharmacist must be convinced beyond a peradventure that he releases such information only to those authorised to request it.

A problem may arise in a pharmacy after a positive pregnancy test in a minor – under 16 years old. The advice in the PSC's Code of Ethics is to keep the matter confidential, but adds a further sentence:

> Rarely, if the pharmacist believes there may be risk to the life of the girl or her pregnancy, following the receipt of this information, it may be judged necessary to inform a responsible person without the girl's consent.
>
> Where necessary any disclosures and their extent should be recorded on the patient's record.

The question arises as to whether the possibility of the patient going on for a termination may be considered to be a 'risk to her pregnancy'. Do the pharmacist's personal values come into the equation here? An interviewing panel may consider that an interesting question to put to a candidate.

There are some personal, named records kept by pharmacists, which must be released to official bodies on demand. These include the CD register, which legally must be available to a whole raft of inspectors, including those from the Home Office and the Pharmaceutical Society.

If they are to be paid for services then pharmacists must keep records and make them available on request to authority inspectors. These include patient medication records, advice to residential homes and a prescription book for the sale of POM. Another possible conflict arises here if the authority demands proof of the provision of a service through sight of identifiable patient records. Must the pharmacist accede to the demand? As in the case of doctors, there is advice that a defence body should be consulted first.

Negligence

Once again the author repeats that he is no legal expert and that readers are advised to take legal advice about such matters when in any doubt. The section following is, as the title of the book says, nothing more than a guide.

We are living in days of increased litigation, fostered by a new generation of the legal profession, which is taking advantage of the relaxed American fashion recently introduced into this country of 'No win, no fee'. Their clients would do well to note, mind you, that there is nothing there to say how large the fee will be for a win. Certainly it will be large enough to make it worthwhile losing the ones they do lose.

As an aside, many solicitors are now being accused of being ambulance chasers. Nonsense, claimed one writer to the *Daily Telegraph*; judging by all their advertisements in hospital A&E departments, they got there first.

Pharmacists and pharmacies need to know this area of the law in some detail in order to take appropriate precautions. Any worker may make a mistake, which may have serious consequences on another person. This would be a civil liability and every pharmacist, like every doctor, should have professional liability insurance. Make sure that your candidates have that and, maybe, pay their future subscriptions upon their appointment as your superintendent or part-time pharmacist.

Having said that the effect of the error would be a civil liability, there are an increasing number of circumstances where serious, fatal errors may be treated as criminal acts under the manslaughter laws.

But back to the solicitor acting for a complainant who wishes to receive compensation for an alleged personal injury. His client must be able to prove two facts of critical importance:

1 that the pharmacist owed a duty of care and has breached it
2 that damage was caused which was reasonably foreseeable.

It could be said that there may be a failure in the duty of care if any patient who presents a prescription or asks for advice that would reasonably be in the pharmacist's knowledge suffered damages as a consequence of an error in that action. In other words, a pharmacist has a duty to be reasonably competent and fails in that duty if a mistake is made that they should reasonably have been able to avoid.

The legally accepted standard is that of the standard of skill of a reasonably competent pharmacist carrying out the same action. Obviously there will be debate about this on both sides of a negligence case.

Implicit in this is that the pharmacist must have taken appropriate steps regarding continuing his education to at least the standards of his colleagues.

As for the damage caused, that is legally the damage caused by the action of the pharmacist despite any pre-existing condition. An example would be that, so far as damages are concerned, it does not matter that the asthmatic patient may have come to no harm from the mistaken dispensing of a beta-blocker if he had not got asthma. The patient did have asthma and did come to harm as a result of the β-blocker dispensed. The error should not have been made in the first place.

In order not to make the error it is the duty of the pharmacist to take reasonable care (the care expected from other pharmacists carrying out the same action, remember) to:

• be sure that the prescription is correctly dispensed
• warn of the dangers of the medicine
• advise the correct dosage.

Often, however, the mistake is made due to some flaw in the system within the pharmacy. The pharmacist should constantly examine and update his pharmacy dispensing operating procedures.

Correct dispensing

If the pharmacist has any doubt whatsoever about what is written on a prescription form, be it printed or in handwriting, then the prescriber should be contacted. That will, of course, be simpler from an in-house pharmacy. That doubt may arise due to the pharmacist's knowledge of the medicine written on the prescription or of his knowledge of the patient. It is the duty of the pharmacist to the patient to be sure.

Warnings

Increasingly, manufacturers are printing warnings on patient medication packs and leaflets. It may be construed as negligence if the pharmacist removed the leaflet or obscured the information on the pack with his own label. It may also be considered negligence, and against his terms of service, if a chemist dispensed a parallel imported pack where neither the warnings nor the leaflet were in English and were, therefore, unintelligible to the patient.

In Appendix 9 the *British National Formulary* carries an exhaustive recommended list of the wording of cautionary and advisory labels and the situations in which they must be used. There is also a comprehensive list of medications with an indication of which warning must be used in which case. The pharmacist is obliged to ensure the appropriate warnings are on his label and the container.

Suggestions about a contract of employment for a pharmacist

It falls upon me, once again, to advise that a legal expert be employed when drawing up any contract of employment. I am merely attempting to give some guidance.

Employment law is a very complex subject and the basis of much litigation, expensive in its implementation and the damages arising from the ignorance of it.

The Employment Rights Act 1966 is the basis of most contracts and it obliges an employer to give a written contract within two months of the employee taking up his position. Despite this, any contract may be varied at any time with the agreement of both parties, except possibly the new pharmacy and the new medical contracts with government which the government can vary unilaterally after 'consultation'.

Every contract must contain the following information:

- the name and address of the employers
- the name and address of the employee
- the date of commencement of employment
- the salary, frequency of payment and method of calculating it
- the agreed hours of work
- the agreement regarding holiday entitlement, pay etc
- the sickness and sick pay agreement
- the pension terms
- the job title or description
- the notice to be given by either side to terminate employment.

In addition to that, it is the duty of every employer to ensure that every employee is given:

- details of disciplinary measures
- a counsellor within the firm with whom to discuss disciplinary matters and grievances
- contracting out details.

The question arises, who does the employee superintendent pharmacist have as a counsellor? Possibly one of the professional bodies – the PSNC, the LPC, NPA or the Pharmaceutical Society, perhaps?

Having said all the above, the law does not demand that the contract must be a totally written contract. Verbal agreements may also be a part of it.

Both employees and employers have duties under a contract of employment.

Employees' duties

- To turn up for work and follow the terms of the contract.
- To be reasonably competent and not negligent.
- Within lawful reason, to do as they are asked by the employer or a superior.
- Not to damage the employer's property.
- To act in good faith. By which this means, not to commit fraudulent acts or, in the case of a pharmacy, not to break confidentiality – among other matters.

Failure to observe these could be taken as a breach of contract by the employee.

Employer's duties

- To provide wages, sick pay and other agreed payments.
- To follow the EC Working Time Directive.
- To trust the employee.
- To provide a safe working environment.
- To allow time off for some employees to carry out public functions, e.g. a mayor.
- To repay genuine expenses incurred in the job.

Any failure to observe these obligations could be taken as a breach of contract by the employer and may be the cause of litigation on the grounds of constructive dismissal, in some cases.

A safe working environment

By definition pharmacies contain large quantities of potentially lethal medications, poisons and other noxious substances. It could fairly be expected that a superintendent pharmacist would be more aware of this than anybody, but other employees may not be.

However, the pharmacist will in most cases be an employee of the firm and the firm is responsible to the obligations in the *Control of Substances Hazardous to Health Regulations 1988*, even in the case of the pharmacist.

A hazardous substance is any substance which in above-normal amounts may cause a hazard to human health. The employer must:

- determine the risk involved and the precautions needed
- introduce precautionary measures and train employees about them
- make sure that the precautions are being followed.

The owners of a pharmacy would be breaking the Regulations if they did not provide safekeeping, for instance, for poisonous substances.

Other matters

Other matters relating to Employment Law are discussed in Chapter 4.

Finally about pharmacists

Much of what is written above about the duties and terms of pharmacists may well be torn up by the Shipman Enquiry team on publication of their report in 2004. They will be especially concentrating on CDs, their prescription, keeping, dispensing, record keeping and destruction.

Dame Janet Smith, Chairman of the Shipman Enquiry Team, hopes to 'close the audit trail loop' to allow monitoring of CDs from manufacturer to wholesaler, pharmacy, patient and back to the pharmacy for destruction.

How to find a pharmacist

It has been said that there are fewer people interested in pharmacy as a career at any level than ever before — so few, in fact, that, as for GPs, it has been necessary for the NHS to trawl the world for recruits. However, the obvious way to start in this country is to put an advertisement in your local paper, but there are alternatives. The following list may be helpful.

- Place an advertisement in:

  - the local papers
  - the national papers — *The Times, Daily Telegraph, The Guardian, Independent*
  - *The Chemist & Druggist*
  - *The Pharmaceutical Journal.*

- Find advertisers in the above pharmacy magazines.
- Find an agency such as:

  - The Pharmacy Relief Staff Agency, 2 Crown Court, Sturton-le-Steeple, Near Retford, Nottingham, DN22 9HX www.pharmacyrelief.co.uk
  - Pharmacy Locums UK www.pharmacylocumsuk.com
  - Em Recruitment www.emrecruitment.co.uk
  - ETI Recruitment 01332 768888
  - Reed Health Professionals www.reedhealth.co.uk 0121 616 3981.

Alternatively, search the internet through Google, for instance, by inputting the field 'Pharmacy Employment' or a similar wording.

On the other hand, if you are opening a pharmacy using the proposed OFT deregulation mechanism, it is possible that a high-street pharmacist working for a multiple may see the warning signs and volunteer to join your enterprise.

Having found a suitable superintendent pharmacist and a part-time pharmacist if one is needed, it is now time to look for other members of staff, the dispensary technician and, perhaps a counter assistant.

The pharmacy technician

The importance of the pharmacy technician should not be underestimated, as every dispensing doctor will say. The technicians are the people who will be carrying out the vast majority of the dispensing under the supervision of the pharmacist.

Despite the importance of their job there is still no statutory obligation for them to be either qualified or a member of a recognised professional body. Nevertheless, the original Dispensing Doctors Association (DDA) took the lead in this 20 years ago by instituting a dispensary assistants' course. The Association went on to encourage dispensing practices to employ only qualified staff and that course is still going from strength to strength.

The Pharmaceutical Society is only now recognising the Association of Pharmacy Technicians (APT) as the professional body for these vital employees. I understand it has been a hard fight.

The Association of Pharmacy Technicians

The Association of Pharmacy Technicians was founded in 1952 to further the interests of qualified staff employed in pharmacies. It maintains a list of well over 1000 qualified members nationwide.

On its website the APT provides its mission statement:

> The Association of Pharmacy Technicians UK seeks to both ensure and continually improve upon professional, educational and practice standards for registered Pharmacy Technicians and allied support staff in all healthcare and pharmaceutical organisations. The APTUK will achieve this overall objective through the establishment of open and robust professional regulatory systems.

It then goes on to present the aims of the organisation.

- To maintain, safeguard and enhance the professional and educational standards of all pharmacy technicians.
- To seek registration.
- To improve educational standards (BTEC/SCOTVEC qualification, NVQ/SNVQ National Occupational standards).
- Advising the RPSGB of how technicians can be put to greater use.
- To promote safe and cost effective dispensing, distribution and use of medicines.
- To promote pharmacy technicians as an integral part of the patient care team.

One of those aims has recently been achieved. The Pharmaceutical Society has agreed criteria for entry to a Pharmacy Technicians Register and this will be started on 1 January 2005.

From 2007, only pharmacy technicians with an S/NVQ level 3 in pharmacy services will be permitted to join the Register and to use the protected title – 'pharmacy technician'.

However, for the two years between 1 January 2005 and 31 December 2006, pharmacy technicians without the S/NVQ level 3 in pharmacy services will be allowed to have their names added to the Register.

The large group of technicians who do not hold the above qualification may still be able to join the Pharmaceutical Society's Register if they hold one of the following qualifications:

- BTEC in pharmacy services
- BTEC National Certificate in science or applied science (pharmaceutical)

- London Institute City and Guilds Dispensing Technicians Certificate
- Certificate of the Society of Apothecaries
- Dispensing certificate of the Army or RAF medical corps
- NPA 2-year dispensing technicians correspondence course, pre-1998
- Boots 2-year dispensing training programme, pre-1993.

One notable omission from this list issued by the Pharmaceutical Society is the DDA dispensary technicians BTEC Continuing Education Certificate distance-learning course, developed at Nottingham University Department of Pharmacy. Could this be because the RPSGB opposed the DDA tooth and nail as it developed the course – even to the extent of forbidding pharmacists from helping to improve standards in this way?

Does the Pharmaceutical Society think it reasonable that these well-trained and enthusiastic individuals should be instantly devalued because of its own narrow-mindedness? Far better for the Society to improve cooperation between the professions by examining the course and, if they feel it necessary, suggesting improvements to allow these technicians freedom to move unhindered from a doctor's dispensary to pharmacy if they so wish.

Job description for a dispensary technician

The following is but a brief suggestion for the employer and the superintendent pharmacist to build on.

The main purpose of the dispensary technician is to ensure:

- that the dispensary is properly stocked under the direction of the pharmacist
- that all medicines are dispensed accurately and promptly under the pharmacist's supervision
- that all dispensary equipment is kept in proper order
- that all medicines are kept safely under the pharmacist's direction
- that the dispensary is kept clean and tidy at all times.

The main duties of the dispensary technician are:

- to dispense medicines accurately according to the prescription form and make them ready for checking by the pharmacist
- not to dispense to unauthorised persons without the explicit consent of the pharmacist
- not to dispense at all in the absence of the pharmacist
- to dispense and record private prescriptions and their payments
- to observe all dispensing laws and regulations at present in force
- to keep all necessary records as directed by the pharmacist
- to keep up to date at all times with dispensary practice.

Legal protection for dispensary technicians

The technician's employer is vicariously liable for the actions of his employees. In addition to that, the employer will have liability insurance cover, which includes staff cover so if it comes to suing either the penniless assistant or the well-insured pharmacist, the patient's solicitor will almost certainly choose the pharmacist or his employer – your company.

From the employer's point of view it is obviously extremely important that the dispensary assistant has been properly trained along the lines of any of the above qualifications. It is equally important that dispensing, even in an emergency, is not delegated to untrained counter staff and never takes place in the absence of the pharmacist.

The continuing education of all staff should be a foundation stone of your pharmacy.

Finding a dispensary technician

The following measures may be taken to find a qualified dispensary technician.

* Approach the Association of Pharmacy Technicians UK (www.aptuk.org.uk).
* Advertise in the local press.
* Advertise in the national press.
* Advertise in the medical press.
* Advertise in the pharmaceutical press.
* Look for advertisements in those publications.
* Place notices on hospital noticeboards.

Use an agency such as:

* Jobs in Health www.jobsinhealth
* The Pharmacy Relief Staff Agency, 2 Crown Court, Sturton-le-Steeple, Near Retford, Nottingham, DN22 9HX www.pharmacyrelief.co.uk
* Pharmacy Locums UK www.pharmacylocumsuk.com
* Em Recruitment www.emrecruitment.co.uk.

Use a search engine, such as Google, inputting 'Dispensary technician'.

Rates of pay
It is best to approach the APT for a current up-to-date scale of pay for their members (www.aptuk.org.uk).

Contract of employment
All the employment laws applicable to pharmacists apply to dispensary technicians and all other employees. They have been discussed here and in Chapter 4.

The contract must be presented to the new staff member within two months of the commencement of employment.

Other matters
Remember, if the pharmacy is to be open for six days then at least two technicians will be required.

Always involve the superintendent pharmacist in the interviewing process. Indeed, it would be diplomatic to make him responsible for the appointment of this valuable member of staff. He may even remind you that the Pharmaceutical Society makes him responsible for all the members of his staff and therefore that he must interview all candidates.

Pharmacy counter assistant

This post needs to be filled only if the in-house pharmacy is to sell sufficient OTC medicines and general goods to make it worthwhile. It is for the company directors, the doctors, as owners of the business to make a positive decision one way or the other about that. There are costs, but there are also profits. All the previously described employment laws apply here, too.

It is advisable that the dispensary counter assistant be given some training in the handling of medicines. This should involve the difference between OTC medicines and pharmacy only medicines (P-only). The days of the counter assistant thrusting her hand in the air to gesticulate to a distant pharmacist for permission to sell a P medicine should have long gone. That certainly should be so in the primary care health centre pharmacy discussed here.

There should also be a keen awareness of when to take direct advice from the pharmacist and when and what questions to ask the customer prior to that. To that end the pharmacist should always be approachable by the staff.

It should not be expected that the pharmacy counter assistant be a trained pharmacist or even a dispenser, but they must have more insight and better training, in medicines at least, than an ordinary shop assistant.

To this end the formation of a new association, the Association of Professional Pharmacy Staff (APPS), was announced in late March 2004 by the Communications International Group, the NPA and Precision Database Marketing. The aims of the Association are to:

- achieve public recognition for pharmacy staff
- establish a cohesive forum for structured training
- ensure that training materials are tailored to the needs of pharmacy staff.

Membership of the Association will depend upon candidates undertaking basic training and continued professional development each year. More information was not available at the time of writing but the NPA will be able to help.

Job description for a pharmacy counter assistant

The following are a few suggestions for inclusion in the counter assistant's job description:

- to be willing to undergo basic training and regular updates
- to be aware of the difference between OTC and P-only medications
- to have some basic knowledge of pharmacy law and regulations regarding the sale of these classes of medicines
- not to sell P-only preparations without the direct consent of the pharmacist
- to know when to call the pharmacist for advice and not to be afraid to do so
- to have some awareness of minor human conditions
- not to be tempted to overstep his/her knowledge boundaries
- to serve the customer safely at all times
- to handle prescription forms safely and efficiently by handing them to a dispenser or the pharmacist
- to maintain absolute confidentiality of all information given by patients
- to adopt a professional attitude towards the job

- to keep the pharmacist aware of levels of counter stock
- to keep the working area clean and tidy at all times.

Pay scale

A suggestion is that the pharmacy counter assistant be paid on the local pay scale for shop assistants plus an element to acknowledge the extra training and responsibility involved in the job.

Finding a pharmacy counter assistant

Pharmacy counter assistants may be found through some of the above pharmacy staff agencies plus:

- the local press
- the Job Centre
- local private employment agencies
- retail-worker magazines
- Alchemy 01264 336888
- Eames, Jones & Judge Hawkings 01438 840984.

Staff honesty

One final, hopefully not very relevant, section to this chapter involves the honesty, or the checking of the honesty of the staff.

The pharmacist or the directors may well have known an employee for many years and, in the case of the pharmacist, may have played golf together. But who knows when bad times will come round the corner and debts begin to mount? Just because he seems honest does not mean that circumstances have not changed to make him dishonest. Temptation is a hideous beast that will strike anywhere at anytime. Ensure that security is tight at all times.

Of one thing you may be sure. It is very unlikely that staff dishonesty will be as crude as dipping a hand in the till. After all, most of those are now efficiently computerised and many need the staff member to insert an identity code or use a swipe card before use.

The 'efficient' dishonest staff member will under-ring the till or pretend that some high-value item has been shoplifted. The first the pharmacist may know that something is going on in the busy pharmacy could be when a customer or other staff express their suspicions.

If this is the case then the pharmacist must be very, very careful when investigating the suspicion, and that ought to include, if possible, obtaining a statement from the person who mentioned it. There must be more than just a sus-picion when the member of staff is confronted. It must be possible to prove the offence took place. Without that no disciplinary action can be taken.

During the construction of the pharmacy a security firm will have been consulted (*see* Chapter 8). Return to them with your suspicions – but no names, of course – and ask for their help and advice in tracking down the culprit. They may install miniature CCTV (closed-circuit television) cameras or other gadgetry to obtain evidence. The NPA may also be able to help with advice.

When you believe there is sufficient evidence, seek help from your solicitor and with their support, ask the employee for permission to search them and their locker. Should this confirm the wrongdoing, then a formal disciplinary meeting must be held either under the company rules (of which all employees should have a copy) or the ACAS Code of Practice rules. It is strongly advised that there should always be a third person present as a witness.

The pharmacist should then put forward the case with the evidence and invite the employee to comment. If the case is proven and there are no mitigating circumstances then the appropriate disciplinary action can be taken according to company rules and the employee's contract of employment. Commonly, the first offence generates a warning – written or verbal. This holds for six months.

The employee does, of course, have a right to appeal, in which case a further meeting must be held.

Fraud and theft are, of course, criminal offences and if proven or strongly suspected should be reported to the police.

Beware of being tempted in a fit of anger to summarily dismiss the errant employee. There may have been some legal irregularity in the disciplinary procedure, which could allow the employee to have the case dismissed at a tribunal. That could cost the firm dearly. Everything must be documented carefully.

Prevention is always better than a cure. So it is a good idea to have set company rules, which are well understood by all employees. Among the rules could be informing the staff that the company is aware of all the possibilities for wrong-doing by staff members and is constantly alert to them. They may even be listed in the rules. The NPA suggests that these possibilities include:

* till procedures
* staff purchase/discount register
* ordering goods in the company name but for their own use
* receiving and signing for goods
* the involvement of family members as customers.

All this should be explained to the employee, either before or upon taking up employment with the pharmacy. A written copy should be signed by every staff member.

References

1   Royal Pharmaceutical Society of Great Britain. *The Annual Register of Pharmaceutical Chemists*. RPSGB, London.
2   Royal Pharmaceutical Society of Great Britain. *The Code of Ethics for Pharmacists*. RPSGB, London.
3   *The NHS (Pharmaceutical Services) Regulations 1992, No. 662 – Amendments to 1999 (Control of Entry) Regulations*. Stationery Office, London.
4   British Medical Association and The Pharmaceutical Society (published twice yearly) *British National Formulary*. BMJ Books, London.
5   Department of Health (updated regularly) *The Drug Tariff*. Stationery Office, London.
6   Royal Pharmaceutical Society of Great Britain. *The British Pharmacopeia*. RPSGB, London.

Chapter 8

Fitting it out

Everything in this chapter can be regarded as a skeleton to be fleshed out with other ideas from a series of experts. It is not a definitive work but it should be enough to get the project moving along the right lines.

The first consideration should be for the staff. They should be provided with a suitable rest room where their outside clothes may be stored and where they may take their break periods or eat their lunches. Also in this area should be a staff toilet, hand-washing and tea-making facilities with cupboards and a refrigerator.

It may be possible to save valuable space by sharing toilet, washing and rest facilities with health centre staff. This will have the big advantage of integrating the pharmacy staff with everybody else.

That apart, the modern pharmacy has three main purposes:

1   to dispense medicines – NHS and private – safely and efficiently
2   to permit confidential consultations
3   to retail OTC medicines and whatever general goods may be compatible with a pharmacy.

The first important decision to be made is which of these three functions the in-house pharmacy will be undertaking. Of the three, only one may be taken for granted – the dispensing of medicines – and, of course, every pharmacy has to be efficiently fitted out for that.

If there is space then it is recommended that a small area be set aside, especially in your in-house surgery, where confidential consultations may be had with patients by the pharmacist. This is probably more useful here than in the high-street pharmacy where the pharmacist may not have easy access to a doctor for advice over difficult problems.

An early decision needs to be made as to what, if anything, the pharmacy will retail. If the pharmacy is little more than a converted room in a health centre, then it is not likely that there will be much space to sell anything other than OTC medicines. OTCs are essential, but care should be taken in choosing which ones to stock (that will be covered in Chapter 10).

If the pharmacy is developed in tailor-made premises added on to the health centre then, as they say, the world is your oyster. Visit several pharmacies in the towns to get some idea of the goods that they believe, from their presence on their shelves, to be profitable. Again, more of this in Chapter 10.

The new dispensary

What may be considered ideal? Unfortunately, there may be many in-house companies that have little choice. They will have to make the best use of the space or room that they have. To do that, pause for a little thought before knocking down walls and slamming up shelves. Think what the purpose of the dispensary is. It is not simply to count out pills and hand them over the counter.

Many other activities go on there, including: the safe storage of medicines, controlled drugs and poisons; record-keeping; computing; mixing medicines; washing; cleaning; and, increasingly, the writing of repeat prescriptions. Other activities will be mentioned as the chapter goes on.

Whether the pharmacy is started from scratch in a new-build or having to make the best out of existing premises, it is vital to ensure that the superintendent pharmacist is, if possible, involved in the planning from the very beginning. After all, who knows better than the pharmacist how to lay out the dispensary? And, of course, the Pharmaceutical Society throws some responsibility on the pharmacist for the premises in which all the staff work.

The structure

One of the most important parts of any dispensary is not the pill counter or the computer system, but the security precautions.

Security

Some years ago when writing about the design of the dispensing doctor's dispensary in an earlier book, *The Complete Dispenser*,[1] I commented, somewhat bluntly:

> Unfortunately we live in a society plagued with parasitic, destructive, thieving drug addicts so the prime consideration for any dispensary, new or old, is security and this begins with the structure of the premises. Their targets are fourfold: drugs, prescription forms, cash and computer equipment.

These days those words would not be considered very PC but it is unfortunate that they still hold true. If anything, the situation has worsened and will continue to do so while ever the politicians tinker with the drug laws.

There is no doubt that it is far easier to build or design-in security than to add it later, so at an early stage call for the help of the district crime prevention officer (CPO) of the local police. He should be a mine of information and advice. Not least important of the advice will be which security firms are trustworthy and effective. Try to get three names and follow that up with three interviews and estimates or tenders for the work to be done. Then have all the work carried out together.

The dispensary will, by definition, contain a multitude of poisonous, addictive or simply dangerous products. The law demands that controlled drugs be kept in a locked steel cabinet, bolted to the wall or floor within the dispensary. So, think of this as an analogy for the dispensary as a whole, that is, as a secure, locked container that may be isolated from the rest of the primary care centre.

Pay strict attention to the building to prevent unauthorised access from any direction. That means considering the doors, windows, ceilings, walls and the outside of the premises.

- *Doors* – Every internal door to the dispensary must be security lockable and of sound structure rather than soft ply or veneer. The outside door is of particular interest and as it may also be the door of the health centre it should be safe to assume that it is already secure. If not, why not?
- *Windows* – If there are any windows then they must be of sound structure, lockable, alarmed and possibly barred or shuttered. It is useful to have a central security locking system, which involves all doors and windows when the premises are vacated.

  Only the small, upper part of divided windows should be openable and that by a limited amount. Louvred windows are unsuitable as the louvres may be readily removed from the outside. Finally, it could be worthwhile giving some consideration to hardened glass.
- *Walls* – The important criterion about the walls of the premises is that none of them should be made of a soft, partition structure. Just remember what the dispensary will contain. Controlled drugs are in a steel box for safety, so make the walls, the equivalent to the box, equally strong by using a hard building material such as brick or concrete blocks. A builder will be able to give advice about this.
- *Ceiling* – It may well be above eye-level, but it should not be above consideration. The author had a dispensing practice for over 25 years and twice during that time burglars lifted roof tiles and entered the dispensary by cutting a hole in the ceiling. Unusual, maybe, but it is worth thinking about.
- *Throughout* – Passive infrared (PIR) or some equivalent alarm sensors should be placed at strategic points throughout the pharmacy as a whole. In addition to them it could be called neglectful, under the Health & Safety at Work Regulations, not to have strategically placed panic buttons for the staff – see below.

  The entire pharmacy must be protected by a modern security alarm system directly connected to a central control, which will warn both the police and the owners or the security company control, if it is triggered by an intruder. Instantaneous ringing at 'control' with a delay at the premises to permit the police to apprehend the culprit is a very useful facility. It is also useful to have a keypad entry code that allows a staff member under duress to open the premises and alarm 'control' without triggering the premises alarm.
- *Staff security* – It is a sad fact of life that even medical and pharmacy premises are frequently attacked by unpleasant members of society. Pharmacies and dispensing practices are particularly targeted because they are thought to contain scheduled drugs and cash.

  Early in 2004 seven PCT managers offered their support to pharmacists whose staff or themselves had suffered a series of robberies or knife attacks. The PCTs recommended:

  - fast fax links between the pharmacy and the local police station in an attempt to gain a fast response from the police
  - extending zero-tolerance schemes to pharmacies
  - improved funding for improved security

– training for pharmacists and staff on the handling of aggressive patients
– efficient siting of 'panic buttons'.

Pharmacy security is being taken seriously by politicians these days. The Conservative Shadow Health Minister has suggested that pharmacy security should be the same as that of Post Offices. He believes there should be roll-down shutters, video cameras and the full cooperation of the police.

* *Outside the premises* – Let's face it, every intruder must, by definition, come from the outside, so it is very sensible to attempt to prevent entry as well as to detect it when entry has been forced. Pay serious attention to the outside of your premises.

Remembering my experience, that should include the roof. If the pharmacy is but one part of a very large 'one-stop' primary care centre it may be too expensive to strengthen the entire roof, but it may not be impossible to prevent or deter access to it in some way.

Other measures which may be considered could include:

– steel roller blinds on the windows and doors
– outside alarms bells, CCTV systems and PIR or light-level controlled security lighting.

Many security experts consider continuous floodlighting to be more efficient than intermittent, sensor controlled lighting.

Exposed security items such as the ones above may need themselves to be protected from tampering or vandalism. That includes exposed telephone lines upon which security systems depend.

Burglary is not the only danger to which the premises are exposed. An increasing number of the young seem to get a buzz out of setting fire to premises – any premises which are not protected. Most of the above will go some way to deter arsonists but, as simple common sense, do not leave piles of flammable waste material around the outside of the building. Inside the building some consideration may be given to a sprinkler system and, of course, smoke alarms connected to the security centre.

Useful security contacts

There are a number of national security firms and even more local outfits, some of which may, just may, be cowboys. Ask your crime prevention officer for advice to help sort them out. You may also get some help from local shopkeepers or dispensing practices.

Inclusion on the list does not imply any recommendation – nor the reverse.

* the local CPO
* the police architectural liaison officer
* The fire prevention officer (FPO)
* The Alarms Inspectorate & Security Council; 01704 500897
* The Security Systems and Alarms Board; 0191 296 3242
* The Association of Security Consultants; 07071 224 865; www.security consultants.org.uk
* The National Security Inspectorate; www.nsi.org.uk.

At the same address is:

- Pharmacy Mutual Insurance Co Ltd; 01727 844344
- Pharmaceutical and General Provident Society.

Presumably the more precautions taken by the pharmacy the lower the premium.

Other useful contacts

Inclusion in this list does not imply a recommendation.

Burglar alarms
- Chubb Alarms Ltd; 0800282494
- Modern Security Systems Ltd; 01442 234123.

Fire alarms
- Chubb Alarms Ltd; 0800 282494
- Photain Controls plc; 01903 721531.

Fire extinguishers
- Firemaster Extinguisher Ltd; 0207 852 8585
- First Aid Supplies; 0208 443 1123.

CCTV
- Case Security Ltd; 01727 846645; www.casesecurity.co.uk
- ITC; 01708 725511
- Modern Security Systems Ltd; 01442 234123
- White Group; 0113 274 4811.

Security locks
- Aardee Spring Lock Co; 0141 553 2070
- Yale Security Products; 01902 366911.

Security systems
- Case Security Ltd; 01727 846645; www.casesecurity.co.uk
- Chubb Alarms Ltd; 0800 282494
- Esselte Meto Ltd; 01344 701200
- ITC; 01708 725511
- Pilkington UK Ltd; 0113 249 7511
- Yale Security Products; 01902 366911.

Fixtures and fittings

Right, then, the shell of the pharmacy is complete and the premises are secure so now let us furnish it with fixtures, fittings, equipment and all the rest of the appurtenances of the efficient pharmacy.

The first piece of advice is to include your superintendent pharmacist in all the design stages.

The second piece of advice is to visit as many pharmacies in nearby towns as possible. If you go along with your pharmacist and introduce yourself as the owner of a new pharmacy in some other town, you may even be able to persuade the pharmacist to show you around but, on the other hand, perhaps not. These visits will give an impression of the size, fittings and layout for your own pharmacy.

The third piece of advice is to sit down and work out what the dispensary functions will be. The following may be a help here. The dispensary will be used for:

* mixing and dispensing medicines
* keeping records and used prescriptions
* selling and ordering of medicines
* the secure storage of medicines, poisons and other products.

Storage

Storage will be needed for a multitude of items:

* medicines of all kinds – including controlled drugs and poisons
* refrigerated items
* containers of all kinds
* measuring and mixing apparatus
* prescriptions
* reference books
* poisons.

Counter space

Be as generous as space allows. It may not be possible to add more later and counter space has a long list of uses, amongst which are the following:

* writing
* computer systems and printers
* prescription transactions – script reception
* pill counting – even in these days of patient packs
* mixing and weighing extemporaneous items, where requested
* holding completed prescription orders
* washing and cleaning – a double-sink unit
* telephones.

It is worth bearing in mind that patients may request their repeats immediately, but collect them two days or a week later or, incredibly, sometimes they never collect their medicines. Some holding space is necessary.

All counters must be made of an easily cleanable material.

Dispensary designers

It is at this stage that specialist dispensary designers should be called in. It has been said that the three most important objectives in dispensary design are:

1   creating time for counselling
2   creating time and space savings
3   turning walking time into counselling time.

To these I would add the even more important objective:

4   the safe and efficient dispensing of medicines.

Note the emphasis on counselling in today's pharmacy where a high proportion of the actual dispensing of medicines is carried out by the technicians. This is so that the pharmacist may be released to carry out the increasing number of new roles considered appropriate for the pharmacist by today's politicians.

Pharmacies are very labour-intensive – labour accounting for around 70% of dispensary costs – so it is important to reduce wasted effort to a minimum. The efficient storage and handling of dispensary products will create time and space savings, which may be used to allow time for consultations and the space in which to hold them.

The effects of increasing efficiency can be illustrated by some figures. The minimum distance walked to make up a prescription in one dispensary under survey was 49 feet and the maximum 86 feet with an average of 67 feet. A redesign reduced the maximum to 45 feet – 48% less and the average to 33 feet – 50% less.

Using 300 prescriptions a day as an example, the reduction in walking distance[3] was worked out at 715 miles – yes, miles – a year. Translate this into time saved and it amounts to an astounding 13 working weeks, which could be put to other, more profitable uses.

A few years ago a paper[4] in *Pharmacy 2000* discussed how dispensaries may be made more efficient simply by analysing stock usage rates to facilitate:

1   stock storage planning so that the most dispensed products are closest to the dispensing point, thus reducing stock selection times
2   minimisation of the floor space used for stock storage
3   the orderly flow of products to the dispensing point by eliminating ad hoc frequent little order refilling of dispensing point stock holdings
4   the gearing of dispensary stock levels to dispensing volumes thus minimising stock holding of slow moving items and highlighting the opportunities to bulk buy dispensary stock if volume discounts are available
5   the systematic storage of dispensary bulk buys, and thus the time efficient movement of the product from bulk storage to the dispensing point stock storage.

An analysis of the 1133 items carried in the subject dispensary found that 111 were classified as 'high volume', 204 as 'Medium volume' and 818 as 'slow volume'.

Slow volume products were defined as those being dispensed less than three times a month and, of these, 334 were dispensed less than twice in three months.

These figures highlight the undoubted fact that the obvious – simple A to Z storage of drugs on shelves – may be far from the most efficient way of going about the job.

In the interest of dispensing efficiency all these slow volume items may be stored furthest from the point of dispensing. There will be three advantages to isolating slow movers:

1   increasing dispensing efficiency
2   reducing stock levels and, thus, storage space
3   increasing the ease of checking of expiry dates.

The *Australian Journal of Hospital Pharmacy* carried an editorial[5] saying that: '...
pharmacists overwhelmingly indicated that they thought the risk of dispensing
errors was increasing'.

It concluded that there was an immediate need to implement systems that
would improve dispensing accuracy. A little later in this chapter there is a discussion of a number of shelving systems with just that in mind.

An efficient dispensary designer will take all this into account and will draw four
sets of plans relating to four stages in the development of the dispensary:

1   the floor plan
2   the construction plan including heating and ventilation
3   the electrical plan
4   the lighting plan.

These will be followed by the finished plan and all should be demonstrated with
the aid of computer 3-D 'walk-through' demonstrations of the designs. Some
designers will follow the job through to completion where others will suggest
subcontracting the shelving and cabinets to specialist manufacturers. In order to
make the greatest ergonomic savings a good motto would be to make the
equipment conform to the design, rather than the other way around.

Design consultants

In the case of major projects such as this it is vital to approach at least three
consultancies in the early stages. As in the previous lists, the appearance of a
company in the following list is not necessarily a recommendation.

- AMEC Construction Ltd; 01789 204288
- JR Furnishing Contracts Ltd; 01480 811420
- Medical & Scientific Structures Ltd; 01904 610643
- PA Consulting Group; 01763 261222
- Tanvec Ltd; 01252 703663.

The National Pharmaceutical Association service
The NPA has a planning and design service for members. For what they call 'a
competitive fee', they will visit the premises to discuss what they see as your
needs and make recommendations on how to achieve them. The visit will last for
three hours and the fee is non-refundable.

The second stage of the NPA service is to design and carry out the entire project
of getting the new pharmacy up and running. Appropriate builders and shopfitters
are approached for quotations and advice is given about the best designs.

A major benefit is that their fees may be refundable if an NPA-approved
shopfitter is chosen and the NPA planning department is told of this in advance.
In any case the fees include monitoring and following through the project from

beginning to end. The NPA can be contacted at: NPA 38–42 St Peter's Street, St Albans, Herts AL1 3NP; 01727 832161.

It is all very well to trust the experts, but it is helpful to have at least an inkling of what is needed yourself before calling them in. The following pages will give some guidance.

Power supply

Electrical sockets are needed in some profusion as there will be many items of equipment depending on their efficient provision:

- the computer and printer(s)
- a fax machine, possibly
- a pill counter
- mixer/blender
- refrigerator
- vacuum cleaner/polisher

. . . to mention a few.

Lighting

It is important here that the designer takes note of the Workplace (Health, Safety and Welfare) Regulations and avoids shadows in work areas and makes sure that light penetrates effectively into cupboards to avoid inadvertent loss of stock and equipment. Light switches should be placed in the most convenient positions.

Emergencies

The essential 'panic button' must not be forgotten and should be strategically placed where any member of staff may get at it. Could this be connected to other security devices such as roller blinds, door locks and alarms?

Shelving and stock storage

The first thing to know here is that there are almost as many systems as days in the month and not all of them involve shelves. Have a look at as many as possible and consult closely with your designer.

The carousel
There is a very efficient revolving carousel system, which allows the dispenser to have the stock in the immediate vicinity of the dispensing counter without the need to walk all those extra miles. Many GPs will recognise a similar system which they use for medical records. In each case, the dispenser or receptionist turns around from the counter and spins the carousel until the appropriate item or set of notes comes to the front.

The carousel comes in two sizes – 180 cm and 110 cm diameter – each with 10 extendable sloping shelves for restocking at the rear to permit first in, first out stock rotation.

The 180 cm version provides easy access to no less than 50 metres of shelving without the dispenser having to do anything other than turn around.

The use of this system has shown that dispensing times may be cut by 50% with greatly reduced dispenser fatigue and risk of errors. If your dispensary is of limited size then it is well worth consideration for your high and medium volume stock.

StockFlow

The StockFlow system is a free-standing modular range of storage units with interchangeable shelves, trays and drawers. It is designed to make the best use of available space.

Once again the trays are sloping and extendable for restocking at the rear to permit efficient stock rotation as picked items allow the stock to slide forwards.

Rombic

This is an unusual looking system consisting of a vertical bank of around 20, 1-metre long, moderately deep, metal drawers with the fronts sloping downwards from left to right to allow stock to slide sideways to facilitate usage and stock control. Banks of drawers may be arranged side by side.

Further information

Further information about these systems may be obtained from: Sintek Ltd, 44 Cobden House, Cobden Street, Leicester, LE1 2LB; 0116 253 0818.

Alternative systems

Wall shelves are, of course, the simplest form of storage although, as we have seen, may not be the most efficient. Being the simplest they are often the cheapest as they may be made by local joiners or craftsmen. When estimating the amount and type needed pay attention to pack sizes, container sizes, the need not to 'lose' stock behind other items and the limitations of human height.

There are many other variations on the theme of pull-out, sliding shelf systems and details of these may be obtained from the following suppliers:

- AB Shelving & Design Ltd; 0208 337 4969
- Barlow Shopfitting Ltd; 0114 255 6331
- City Design Ltd, Leicestershire
- Exdrum Storefitters, King Charles Business Park, Heathfield, Devon, TQ12 6UT
- Frederick Moore, 39 Cooks Meadow, Edlesborough, Beds, LU6 2RP
- Pearson & Jefferies, The Old Bakery Workshop, 23 Downend Road, Kingswood, Bristol, BS15 1RT
- Martex Shopfitting; 01392 216606
- KH Woodford & Co Ltd; 01202 396272
- Yorkline Ltd, Seacroft Industrial Estate Leeds, LS14 2AW; 01532 734721
- ZAF Shopfitters Ltd, Nottinghamshire; 0115 975 3551
- Zenith Interiors; www.zenithinteriors.ltd.uk.

The list is by no means exhaustive and, once again, inclusion does not imply recommendation.

Special storage conditions

At this early stage special attention must be paid to the conditions necessary for the storage of particular items. These include temperature-sensitive preparations, controlled drugs and poisons.

Temperature-sensitive drugs – If temperature sensitive items are not correctly stored then apart from the effect of deteriorating drugs on the patient – there may also be the consequences of product liability claims.

The manufacturer will state the recommended storage conditions on the pack, so examine all containers or the data sheets for storage instructions and keep the drugs at a steady temperature. Temperature instructions indicate:

- 2°–8°C = needs refrigeration
- 8°–15°C = needs a cool place
- 15°–25°C = room temperature will suffice.

A sensitive maximum and minimum thermometer should be kept within the refrigerator and a daily record must be kept of its readings. See page 121 for details of a professional pharmacy refrigerator.

Controlled drugs

It is a legal requirement that scheduled drugs must be kept in an approved steel, lockable cabinet bolted to the wall or floor and that a CD register be kept. The suppliers of these cabinets include:

- Phoenix Healthcare Distribution Ltd; 0121 4333030
- Case Security Ltd; 01727 846645; www.casesecurity.co.uk
- William G Fuller; 01424 426094
- Portasilo Ltd; 01904 624872
- James Spencer & Co; 01535 272957
- TMS; 01635 276067; www.tmsuk.net.

Poisons

These must all be kept in a secure, locked cupboard or storage system with access available only by the pharmacist. As previously mentioned, a record must be kept of the movement of all poisons.

It is far easier to build these items in during the design stage than to find some space at a later date.

It is not very likely that a primary care health centre pharmacy will have much call for poisons and, in any case, ordering and delivery may be very speedily arranged.

The dispensary computer

The choice of a dispensary computer system will be covered in some detail in Chapter 9. At this stage, however, the designer will be aware of its existence and that, being a heavily used item, it should be placed in the most ergonomically suitable position with appropriately placed electrical and telephone outlets – and good lighting.

The actual computer and the various keyboards, monitors and printers may well be in separately convenient positions and will therefore need wiring connections to the computer. The computer will be largely used for the production of labels for containers and packaging, stock ordering and control. In the near future there is likely to be a direct link between the pharmacy and the PPA office for the instant transmission of prescriptions for payment and other purposes. In many cases there is already a link between the surgery and the pharmacy and, in the case of this in-house pharmacy, there certainly will be. Having said that, prescriptions can only be 'directed' to a particular pharmacy with the specific, written permission of the patient. That should not be difficult to obtain.

Other dispensary equipment and suppliers

Autoclaves

Every item that is used for the mixing and manufacture of extemporaneous medicines should be kept in a clean and preferably sterile condition. I am uncertain how many pharmacies actually have an autoclave or how much extemporaneous dispensing will be carried out – probably not much in these days of increased litigation and product liability. However, some pharmacies may be so equipped and an in-house pharmacy may use the surgery autoclave. However, just in case, here is a short list of suppliers:

- Baskerville (Reactors & Autoclaves) Ltd, Lancashire; 0161 881 1540
- Phoenix Healthcare Distribution Ltd; 0121 4333030
- Prestige Medical, Lancashire; 01254 682622
- Rodwell Scientific Instruments, Essex; 01268 286646.

Sterilisers

The same comment applies to sterilisers.

- HW Andersen Products Ltd; 01255 428328
- Casbert Pharmaceutical Equipment Ltd; 01782 332511
- Prestige Medical; 01254 682622.

Balances

- Hogg Laboratory Supplies; 0121 233 1972
- Salter Weightronix; 01638 664434.

Tablet counters

Even in these days of almost universal patient packaging there is bound to be a use for such a machine and no dispensary should be without one.

- King Ltd; 01932 565191
- Kirby Devon Ltd; 01752 881717.

Refrigerators

This is a subject worthy of special consideration because a domestic refrigerator is not suitable. It is very likely that it will not maintain the accurate, steady temperature control that is vital for the safe-keeping of so many pharmaceutical preparations and vaccines.

Household refrigerators are designed to keep their contents between 0°C–10°C. A small difference, but zero is freezing and freezing deactivates vaccines, and 10 degrees may effect their potency.

A professional pharmacy refrigerator should be purchased. Thousands of pharmacies will not pay the high price but, as the NPA comments, they are risking both their stock and their patients.

Professional refrigerators are calibrated and factory-set to maintain their internal temperature at the RPS standard of between 2°–8°C throughout the cabinet. They have a built-in digital thermometer, readable from the outside and an alarm that sounds if the temperature varies. The most sophisticated refrigerators keep a record of temperature variations over a specified period of time.

A final comment about the refrigerator. Do not use it for anything other than pharmaceutical preparations – no food or milk!

- Boro Labs Ltd; 0118 981 1731
- Vindon Scientific Ltd; 01457 876616
- Lec Medical; 01243 863161.

Hand-washing unit

All dispensers and pharmacists must ensure scrupulous hygiene and, therefore, must frequently wash their hands. It will be a waste of time to go to the rest room on each occasion, so a hand-washing unit in the dispensary could be helpful.

- Associated Metal (Stainless) Ltd; 0141 551 0707
- Syspal Ltd; 01952 883188.

Waste disposal

There will, inevitably, be some waste apart from returned drugs and medicines. These, of course, must be carefully disposed of as described in Chapters 4 and 10. Other waste may be handled by the local authority or specialist firms.

- Cannon Hygiene Ltd; 01524 60894
- Daniels AC & Co Ltd; 01442 826881
- Northern Incinerators Ltd; 01743 368134
- DOOP Services; 01491 612267.

Hygiene

The dispensary must be a clean environment in order that dispensing be carried out safely.

- protective clothing:
  - Comfy Products; 01262 676417
  - Simplantex Healthcare Ltd; 01424 854566

- cleaning equipment:
  - Hygiene Systems Ltd; 01992 460698
  - Vileda LP; 01274 851104

- hygiene equipment:
  - Self Serve Hygiene Ltd; 0208 941 3033
  - Syspal Ltd; 01952 883188.

Other basic pharmacy supplies

Pharmacies are, primarily, dispensers of medicines and pills and to carry out that duty need some basic supplies:

Bottles – glass

- Beatson Clark plc; 01709 828141
- International Bottle Company Ltd; 01992 551751
- Roma Glass plc; 01473 824405.

Bottles – plastic

- Barclay Stuart Plastics; 01582 726363
- Neken Chemists Supplies; 01482 223424
- International Bottle Co Ltd; 01992 551751.

Closures – child resistant

- Neken Chemist Supplies; 01482 223424
- Rexam Containers Ltd; 01705 370102
- FW Richardson Ltd; 0208 801 6077.

Closures – plastic

- Invicta Plastics; 0116 272 0555
- Regina Industries Ltd; 01782 565646
- Robinson Plastic Packaging; 01623 752869.

Caps – plastic and screw

- FW Richardson; 0208 801 6077.

Tablet cartons

- BAF Printers Ltd; 0113 243 9788
- Popper Print & Packaging; 01707 336271
- Valley Pharmaceutical Packaging; 0208 304 4711.

Monitored dosage systems

- Surgichem; 0161 406 8710
- Velalink; 0800 243771.

Pharmacy stationery

Every pharmacy has the need for fairly basic stationery – other than headed notepaper, compliments slips and the like.

CD and poisons registers

- Jordan Woodrows Ltd; 0151 207 3000
- Phoenix Healthcare; 0121 4333030.

Patient information leaflets

- Medica Packaging Ltd; 01270 253777.

Pharmaceutical leaflets

- Boardwater Press Ltd; 01707 336271
- Cleanprint; 01638 660063
- Fine Print; 01482 326422.

None of the lists in the above categories is exhaustive. More complete lists may be found in that extremely useful publication, *Chemist & Druggist Directory*.

Confidential consultation area

If your pharmacy and pharmacist are to make the most of this valuable service, then the pharmacist should not hide away in the back of the dispensary. He must be readily seen even when in the dispensary and be easily contacted by the counter assistant. That means that the dispensary itself must be like the bridge of a ship – a command post from which the captain can see everything. It should also have a small private area for making and receiving confidential telephone calls.

There will be many occasions when customers will seek that little bit extra piece of advice, either about their medicines or their health. For this you will need to design-in a confidential consultation area.

Remember what was said earlier, that the dispensary should be designed to save time which may be better used consulting patients. Consultation often means profit.

The area need not be large because only one customer will be using it at a time and it certainly should not be a closed room, because the pharmacist remains in charge of the pharmacy at all times and must not be out of sight.

By definition, the area must be away from other customers and staff so that there is no possibility of embarrassment if sensitive topics are being raised. On the other hand, it must be possible for the staff – but not other customers – to see that a patient is waiting to see the pharmacist. Screening from the shop is essential, either opaque glass or a solid partition, but access must be simple, even for wheelchair users, and clearly signed.

Some considerations for the confidential discussion area could include:

- *Privacy and comfort* – This means that the area should be kept cheerful and attractive at all times, specifically to attract rather than to deter patients. Only if these suggestions are observed will the patient feel less inhibited about revealing problems.
- *Close to the dispensary* – In this way the pharmacist will be able to continue to command the ship without a sensation of pressure. The patient will then get the utmost attention. Thought could be given to installing some system for attracting the pharmacist back to the dispensary.
- *Away from customer areas* – The confidential area could be positioned at the end of the dispensary counter and away from the usual flow of customers around the shop. There must be no chance of a strange customer popping their head around or flapping their ears to see what is going on.
- *Clear signposting* – The signs directing the customer/patient may be suspended from the ceiling at the entrance to the shop with another clear sign close by. Many shy and embarrassed patients would rather walk out than ask. Don't let that happen.
- *Call system* – It is not helpful if the customer arrives at the confidential area and cannot attract attention. An efficient and discrete call system should be installed.
- *The area should be quiet* – It would help lessen the transmission of voices if the immediate walls and floors were of sound-deadening material. From time to time patients may have to wait, so it would be useful to have attractive displays of health promotion material, freely displayed. Display of these items does attract an NHS fee (*see* Chapter 2 on *The Drug Tariff*).[6]
- *Secure storage* – This area will, in some pharmacies, be used by drug addicts coming for their supplies of needles and the filling of their prescriptions. Other patients will ask for diagnostic testing (see below).
- *Computer* – The pharmacist may wish to look up a past record, provide an item of health promotion or supply further information about a medication. It is essential that a terminal of the computer is in this area, together with a printer for appropriate information leaflets and other material.

Diagnostic or 'near-patient' services

An increasing number of pharmacies are being encouraged to carry out diagnostic services for their customers. There is considerable debate about the value and effectiveness of this. Some consider that untutored performance of tests – without counselling by a doctor – can lead to undue distress in the patient. Others believe that pharmacists can be easily trained but, bearing in mind that there is more to doing a test than simply understanding what it is for, that may be unwise. After all, it takes many years to train a GP to that standard, not just a month's correspondence course.

However, more and more pharmacies will be doing it and, more than likely, so will your in-house pharmacy, especially as the pharmacist will have direct and easy access to the GPs for advice or to refer the patient for further help.

There will be a private fee chargeable for every test carried out.

Hypertension

There are many varieties of sphygmomanometer and patients are encouraged to purchase their own. Over the next very few years the old, but accurate, mercury sphygmomanometer will be phased out and replaced by an aneroid or electronic, digital successor. Many pharmacies stock them for sale to their customers.

A professional-looking piece of equipment may be obtained from one of the following suppliers:

* A1 Pharmaceuticals plc; 0207 738 7373
* Braun & Co Ltd; 01652 632273
* Hutchings Healthcare Ltd; 01273 495033.

Cholesterol

Boehringer Mannheim UK Ltd; 01273 480444.

Diabetes

* Boehringer Mannheim UK Ltd; 01273 480444
* MediSense Abbott Laboratories; 01675467044.

Allergy testing

* Imutest; 01492 573900; www.imutest.com.

Other diagnostic equipment

* Bayer plc; 01635 563000
* Cambridge Life Sciences; 01353 667034
* Hypoguard Ltd; 01394 387333
* Seca Ltd; 0121 643 9349.

Ear piercing

Finally, there would seem to be no reason why a pharmacy, especially one capable of sterilising instruments, should not carry out ear-piercing if there are facilities to do so.

* Caflon International Ltd; 01296 434158
* Inverness UK Ltd; 01753 775515.

DIY design?

In case you feel you can do it yourself, with a little help, you may find the following list of contacts helpful.

Dispensary fittings

- E Plan Shopfitting Services Ltd; 01273 517711
- LAZawood; 01883 622151
- RESKA Terrapin Products Ltd; 01908 371001.

Drawer units

- H + H System; 0114 275 6642
- Kardex Systems Ltd; 0208 885 5588
- Link 51 Storage Ltd; 01952 682251.

Lighting

- Concord Sylvania Ltd; 01273 515811
- Crompton Lighting Ltd; 01302 321541
- Thorn Lighting Ltd; 0208 905 1313.

Shelves and shelving systems

- Paul Corbett & Co Ltd; 01732 864004
- RB Shelving Systems UK Ltd; 01234 272717
- Sintek Ltd; 0116 253 0818
- Tebrax Ltd; 01689 897766.

Storage equipment

- Apex Storage Systems Ltd; 01908 561222
- NC Brown (Storage Equipment) Ltd; 01204 596777
- Curver Consumer Products Ltd; 01536 200550
- Profile Systems; 0151 479 3050.

Pharmacy equipment and supplies

- Microclean (Newbury) Ltd; 01635 37901
- Norchem Ltd; 01388 720661
- Nucare plc; 0208 346 8302.

Again, this list is not exhaustive and other suppliers may be found in pharmacy publications.

The retail department

It is very unlikely that this book will be consulted by anybody considering building a large enough pharmacy to contain anything other than a small retail side, so this will be a rather limited discussion of the subject.

This is the front of the house, which should attract customers and make them want to return, time and again. As in most other walks of life, first impressions count for a great deal. A basic principle is to make and keep the place clean and tidy so that shopping will be a pleasant experience, rather than a quick dash in and out.

If your in-house pharmacy does have shop windows, take the trouble to learn something about window dressing, so that they look attractive, but not cluttered.

Pharmacy retailing comes under two headings:

1   general retailing
2   OTC and POM retailing.

It is on this side of the house that two other profitable activities will take place:

1   the consultations and counselling
2   the display of NHS health promotion material.

General retailing

The next time you go into a pharmacy, look very carefully at how the stock and shelving is arranged. If the pharmacist is on the ball and efficient, the advice given in many editions of *Chemist & Druggist* magazine will have been followed over the years and the psychology of retailing will have been carefully considered.

Quick selling, high-profit items will have been carefully displayed so that they become impulse buys as the customer passes to the back of the shop to get to the dispensary. Promotional items will be the first to hit the eye as the customer enters the shop.

To make sales more likely, the shelves and counters will be carefully arranged to make the customer pass them en route to and from the main counter and dispensary. In addition, certain items will be displayed at eye-level to attract the maximum attention. The customer will be subconsciously tempted to take a different route out of the shop to the one taken into it.

The main counter, at the back of the shop, will be where the bestsellers, the high-profit goods and the promotional offers are displayed. Impulse buying is the name of the game.

Hair products, women's and baby products are closely grouped together to help the browsing mother find items she 'needs' for herself. They account for 30% of sales, whereas mens' goods, accounting for a mere 5%, may be found with pharmacy products in an attempt to boost their sale.

The *coup de grâce* is to ensure that the customer has to wait several minutes for the dispensed item. This will ensure pacing the shop, examining the retail goods or having to make a second visit, thus passing through the retail trap a second time.

The only way into and out of any shop is through the door and where better to place a promotional display? Every shopper must pass it and many will be confronted and be attracted to pick up an item on the way to the dispensary.

There is, of course, a great deal more to it than that and it is all very good for business.

Many of the shopfitters listed in this chapter will be pleased to help set up the retail department, but far better to ask your pharmacy designer to help first.

OTC and P-only sales

P-only sales account for, on average, no less than 30% of pharmacy retail sales and OTC preparations – otherwise known as the General Sales List (GSL) – only account for about 10%.

There is absolutely no reason why shoppers should not ask for a particular P-only preparation. To adhere to the law, P-only medications must not be available for customers to pick up themselves, so it will be necessary to have a series of good display cabinets 'behind the counter' or, as an alternative, counter-level displays which are not accessible to them – or both. The specialist shopfitters listed will be able to help here.

It is a legal requirement that these medicines must be sold only under the supervision of the pharmacist and not just under the supervision of the counter assistant. On the other hand, OTC medications may be freely available on accessible shelves.

If your pharmacy is not to sell general goods, but only pharmacy-oriented goods, then some careful consideration to their display should be given.

Now we move on to the fascinating topic of the pharmacy computer system.

References

1   Roberts D (2002) *The Complete Dispenser*. Communications International Group, London.
2   Radio Society of Great Britain (2001) *RSGB EMC Committee leaflets, Radio Transmitters and Home Security Systems EMC 02*. Radio Society of Great Britain, Potters Bar, Hertfordshire.
3   Feros P (1999) Save $35 389 in walking time. *Australian Journal of Hospital Pharmacy*. **29**(3): 176.
4   Smith R (2001) How to increase dispensary stock storage efficiency. *Pharmacy 2000*. **2001**(3): 38.
5   Editorial (2001) Dispensing errors. *Australian Journal of Hospital Pharmacy*. **31**(2).
6   Department of Health (updated regularly) *The Drug Tariff*. Stationery Office, London.

Chapter 9

Pharmacy computing

The modern pharmacy will not be able to function, except at a virtual stone-age level, without an efficient and modern computer system. Long gone are the days, albeit only a dozen or so years ago, when all that was available was the facility to print labels.

Today's pharmacy needs to be in constant contact with the NHS, its own suppliers and the world, as well as carrying out the mundane labelling tasks. Just look at the following list of suggested jobs for the pharmacy computer:

- labelling
- keeping patient medication records – they attract a fee
- stock control and ordering through the wholesaler
- managing the business – VAT, tax, sales and purchases, discounts, etc
- accessing electronic information:
  - CD-ROM
  - local networks, NHSNet
  - from the web
- continuing professional development through the web
- NHS claims for payment – PPA
- future electronic submission of FP10s to the PPA
- emails here, there and everywhere
- direct contact with local doctors, hospitals, other pharmacies
- writing prescriptions for pharmacist prescribing
- designing and printing health promotion leaflets, letters, etc
- electronic point of sale (EPOS).

... and there may well be more added by the month.

So, it is no use going to PC World for this week's bargain system. It just wouldn't cope.

Requirements

Some pharmacists are still using a DOS-based system, with or without Windows, but a new pharmacy should not give this any consideration because suppliers will shortly cease providing support, updates and advancements.

Systems that run on Windows have many advantages, among which is their capability to carry out more than one task at a time. No longer is it necessary to close one program to open another. Letter writing, stocktaking and dispensing may all go on simultaneously, once again saving that vital commodity – time.

Not only that, but while the qualified dispenser is dispensing, the pharmacist may be on the web enhancing his education or, via email, seeking an answer to a query from a colleague. At the same time the PCO may be downloading vital administrative commands for the instant attention of the pharmacist.

Then there is access to the *National Drugs Dictionary* or the *British Pharmacopoeia*, the *British National Formulary* and a myriad of other reference and educational sites all readily online. That is not to mention all the health promotional leaflets waiting to be printed out for the customer.

Add to that the electronic transmission of prescriptions (ETP) to the PPA, when it comes about. Eventually the transmission of electronic health records (EHR) from pharmacy to pharmacy will come along in an attempt to further improve patient care.

None of the above can be accessed through a DOS-based system.

Suppliers

When contemplating the pharmacy system with your superintendent pharmacist, ask the supplier some pertinent questions.

- Can the system dispense whilst connected to the Internet?
- Can it carry out bar code checks whilst other tasks are being carried out?
- Can it run several programs at once?
- Can it stock control whilst dispensing?
- Is there anything it cannot do while dispensing?
- Can it do all the tasks listed and mentioned above?
- Is it NHS-approved?

In short, can it do everything mentioned above – and more?

A respectable supplier, confident with their own product, should be able to give the above information and, in addition:

- the total number of other pharmacy users
- the address of the nearest two or three
- the usage history of the system
- the insurance cost
- staff training facilities and cost
- a full list of 'extras'.

Think carefully about the system and be sure that it has sufficient processor speed, memory (RAM) and a large-capacity hard disc. All these are vital if several tasks are to be carried out together. Make sure that sufficient capacity is built in to allow for the future demands of the NHS and that it complies with the following compulsory standards:

- data protection laws
- NHS standards
- British technical standards
- European technical standards.

The supplier may have an excellent product, but what about their customer support? That is just as important as the machine itself. Make sure that the supplier has satisfactory answers to all the following.

- Is support 24-hours/day, 7 days a week?
- What will this cost?
- How rapid will be the response to a breakdown?
- Is online maintenance and repair available if needed?
- Will spares be instantly available so that downtime is a minimum?
- Can data be recovered?
- Are upgrades a part of the contract?

These are vital questions and demand positive answers.

Labelling

The RPS has laid down minimum standards[1] for labelling in *Guidance on Pharmacy Computer Systems, Medicines Ethics and Practice: A Guide for Pharmacists.*
   The system must be able to produce labels for:

- dispensed medicines
- repackaged medicines – including split packs
- extemporaneously produced medicines
- collection bags for each patient.

All these must be completed according to the Medicines Act, the Society's standards and other legislation.
   There is a standard label size, 70 mm × 36 mm, and printing must be clearly legible without ambiguity and according to standard wording as found in the *Primary Care Drug Dictionary* (www.ppa.org.uk/systems/pcdd_intro.htm). Statutory warnings, as found in the *British National Formulary*[2] (BNF) must be printed in full even if that means two labels need to be used.
   Finally, though unlikely in the in-house dispensary, if more than one dispenser is using the system for more than one patient, the labels should be produced in complete batches for each patient rather than in a haphazard fashion, which may lead to errors.
   There is also a minimum requirement for dispensing, as set out below.
   The database must be comprehensive and include:

- warnings
- dosages
- interactions
- contraindications as in the BNF
- warnings for the pharmacist/dispenser to counsel the patient, if needed.

Updates must be downloaded at least at monthly intervals.
   On a number of occasions pharmacies may not be able to completely dispense a particular prescription to a patient. The computer should allow for this and print appropriate labels, advise the pharmacist to inform the patient and remind that the order must be completed.

Monitored dosage systems (MDS) are sometimes difficult, but the system should be capable of labelling them efficiently and accurately, bearing in mind that they will need far more than one label.

Bar-coded dispensing control

The most modern pharmacy systems allow for the ultimate in safe dispensing, bar-coded control. Each product on the shelf has a unique bar-code on the packaging and in the computer. The generated label will carry a bar-code that is then compared by the wand with the container on the shelf. If the two do not match then the dispensing process should cease. Is this safety feature supported by the system?

Training

As a GP locum working in a succession of practices each, seemingly, with its own computer system, it has been made obvious to me how valuable training would be. As it is, we just learn the basic amount to be able to get by. That is not sufficient if the most is to be made of the system and time is not to be wasted correcting input errors or even computer crashes.

Any reputable systems supplier should have a comprehensive training package for on-site training of all dispensary staff. This must be backed up by both a hard copy manual and a PC- or CD-ROM-based 'Help' module.

Security

Computer security does not simply mean locking or bolting it to the counter. That, of course, would be one way of keeping it, but suppliers such as:

- INMAC, Freepost, Westerly Point, market Street, Bracknell, Berks, RG12 1BS
- MISCO, Faraday Close, Park Farm, Wellingborough, Northants, NN8 3XH
- VIKING DIRECT, PO Box 187, Leicester, LE4 1ZZ
- OFFICE ETC; www.office-etc.com.

carry much more sophisticated items to attempt to ensure that the valuable equipment does not walk out of the dispensary.

But security also involves the security of information and this must be rigorously carried out to comply with the Data Protection Act.

In-house, there are levels of security that allow different users into different parts of the database. The dispenser, for instance, may only need to access the drug list and the patient's previous dispensing history at your pharmacy, but may be barred from the more detailed patient medication records (PMR) and most certainly will be barred from the business details and accounts of the pharmacy.

The superintendent pharmacist will have complete access to the clinical side and to everything else if you have confidence in him to run the business. On the other hand it should be possible to deny access at any level you, the owners, choose. However, to deny any access would breed an atmosphere of distrust.

Then, there is the perennial problem of hackers and viruses. Your supplier should be able to present you with a firewall to prevent unauthorised access.

However, only recently Microsoft let it be known that their most up-to-date versions, including XP, can be accessed by intruders who are able to record a history of every keystroke and thus get hold of confidential personal and business information. The company has said that it is prepared to download protection to Windows' users on request.

Patient medication records (PMR)

The European Standard ENV 13607 demands special standards for these. The records must have the following patient details:

- name, address, telephone number
- sex, date of birth
- NHS number
- GP's name.

The prescriber's details must include:

- name, GMC or NHS GP number
- practice name, address, contact details.

Then come the medication details:

- name
- form, strength, quantity, dosage
- date dispensed.

All the information stored should have originated from the patient and be kept according to the strictures of the Data Protection Act. The system should be able to search data by patient name or NHS number and an additional requirement is that it should be possible to list patients according to nursing home, GP practice or particular medications.

Supplier of software for PMR

- Enigma Health plc; www.enigmahealth.com.

Enigma have recently joined with a company called Dacoll to offer a Saturday call-out service.

Software copies

The pharmacy is burned down together with its computer system or the PC is stolen – so what do you do next? If you do not have a copy of the software and data, all you can do is scream.

Keep secure copies in a safe and separate place out of the building. Take them home at night. Maybe your software supplier will be able to help by providing a secure, encrypted system, which permits the uploading of data every night. On the other hand, the NPA has a disaster recovery service (q.v. page 135).

Erasures

Nothing can ever be permanently erased from a hard disk unless the disk is removed and jumped upon by the proverbial elephant. There will always be an audit trail, as a number of high-profile criminals, including Dr Shipman, found out. So remind your staff that errors cannot be hidden by simply pressing the delete key. It does not work that way.

The Internet and the pharmacist

The Internet carries vast resources of information for pharmacists and their staff and computer-literate people will be able to access most of it with ease. Enormous quantities may be accessed through one of the many search engines such as Google.

Education

Virtually any reference book, textbook or distance-learning course is likely to be accessible through the web. Examples are:

- Electronic Medicines Compendium; www.emc.vhn.net
  This gives details of the product characteristics for licensed medicines. It is updated daily
- *British National Formulary*; www.bnf.org
  The definitive NHS medicines compendium
- Merck Manual; www.merck.com/pubs
  General information on diseases etc
- Medline – the American library of medicine; www.medscape.com
  A complex site of abstracts from around 4000 international medical magazines
- UK medicines information website; www.ukmi.nhs.uk
  An excellent site for medicines information, trials, shortages, new products
- A medicines information service; www.druginfozone.org
  Produced by the London, South East and Eastern Medicines Information service, this site is updated daily. It has been described as a one-stop reference shop.

Magazines
- The Pharmaceutical Journal; www.pharmj.com
- The British Medical Journal; www.bmj.com
- Lancet; www.thelancet.com
- Country Doctor; www.countrydoctor.co.uk
- www.dotpharmacy.com

Evidence-based medicine sites
- National electronic Library for Health; www.nelh.nhs.uk
- Bandolier; www.jr2.ox.ac.uk/bandolier

Other information sites
- Health news; www.health-news.co.uk

Government sites
- www.doh.gov.uk
- www.scotland.gov.uk
- www.wales.gov.uk
- Northern Ireland; www.dhsni.gov.uk
- Medicines Control Agency; www.mca.gov.uk
- National Prescribing Centre; www.npc.co.uk

Pharmacy
- Community pharmacy; www.medicinesmanagement.org.uk; www.managing medicines.com
- Pharmacy in the future; www.rpsgb.org.uk/nhsplan/index
  Designed to help pharmacists make the most of *The NHS Plan* and other papers.
- PSNC; www.psnc.org.uk/database

NPAnet

This site, produced by the NPA, deserves a section of its own. It is designed to serve pharmacy and is secure even though it does have access to the web. The regular features include:

- topical subjects and press releases
- a diary
- drug alerts
- news and archives
- site search
- links to other networks including PSNC and AAH.

There is travel, product and general information in abundance, together with training topics for pharmacists and their staff.

NPA disaster recovery service
Of major importance is a 'disaster recovery service' aimed at pharmacies whose computers have been seriously damaged or stolen. The NPA has created an automated, unmanned process to ensure against data loss. It is sent to the pharmacy by email and regularly backs up, encrypts and transmits the data to a dedicated, secure server. If disaster strikes then data can be recovered from the server within two hours. Access is secure and dedicated to each individual pharmacy and costs around 50p a day.

Another valuable service for pharmacies is the online version of the *Chemist & Druggist Price List*. Subscribers to the magazine have free access to the list.

Suppliers of computer equipment
Computer systems

- AAH Pharmaceuticals; 01928 717070
- Bedford Computers; 01234 271113

- Channel Business Systems; 01444 235236
- Chemtec Systems Ltd; 01772 622839
- Eclipse PMR; 01684 578678
- ECR Retail Systems Ltd; 0208 205 7766
- Enigma/Mediphase; 01932 589904
- GEHIS Ltd; 0121 500 2250
- Park Systems Ltd; 0151 298 2233
- Pharmaceutical Computer Systems Ltd; 0161 941 7011
- Rombus Computers Ltd; 01661 860111.

Computer labelling

- S Calvert Computer Services; 0113 248 4746
- GEHIS Ltd; 0121 500 2250
- Park Systems Ltd; 0151 298 2233.

Computer software

- Bedford Computers; 01234 271113
- Mini Doc Ltd; 01227 788400
- WT Integrated Systems; 01252 703663.

Hardware and software items

- INMAC, Freepost, Westerly Point, Market Street, Bracknell, Berkshire, RG12 1BS
- MISCO, Faraday Close, Park Farm, Wellingborough, Northampton, NN8 3XH
- VIKING DIRECT, PO Box 187, Leicester, LE4 1ZZ
- OFFICE ETC; www.office-etc.com.

Label printers

- Data Label Ltd; 01455 845951
- Esselte Meto Ltd; 01344 701200
- Simpson Label Co. Ltd; 0131 654 2800.

Bar-coding systems

- Cueprint Ltd; 01276 691730
- NOR Systems; 01255 240000.

Point-of-sale systems

- Adart Displays; 01883 652044
- Channel Business Systems Ltd; 01444 235236
- Chemtec Systems Ltd; 01772 622839
- Hadley Hutt Computing Ltd; 01905 795335.

One of these companies, Mediphase, now largely owned by Unichem, claims to have revolutionised pharmacy business systems when it was introduced in 1991. It puts a complex prescription endorsing engine at the heart of its dispensing and patient medication record system (PMR). This ensures that the NHS accurately reimburses pharmacists for the medicines they dispense. Mediphase uses DOS as its computer operating system (OS) and is the pharmacy business system of choice for 4000 pharmacies in the UK.

Mediphase offers the pharmacist a reliable PMR system that ensures accurate endorsement, and:

- accurate endorsing engine
- prints directly onto the prescription
- colour coded navigation
- PMR system
- individual patient record cards
- drug, interactions and doctor inquiry facility
- computer generated labels
- order from major UK wholesalers
- stock control
- oxygen
- DOS-based
- extensive reports.

Note that Mediphase is DOS-based, whereas the future is said to be Windows-based.

Apparently, Mediphase is installed in 4000 pharmacies where it transacts 200 million prescriptions to 14 million patients annually. It should be noted that there are vastly more than 4000 pharmacies in the UK. The suppliers of other systems should be approached.

Useful websites

- Information for health 1998; www.nhsia.nhs.uk/def/pages/info4health/contents.asp
- A spoonful of sugar 2001; www.audit-commission.gov.uk
- Building the information core 2001; www.doh.gov.uk/ipu/strategy/overview
- Delivering IT support for the NHS 2002; www.doh.gov.uk/ipu/whatnew/deliveringit
- PPA; www.ppa.org.uk
- *British National Formulary*; www.bnf.org.

Electronic point-of-sale systems

No discussion of pharmacy or retail computing is complete without mentioning EPOS systems. EPOS is a system used in retailing to provide efficient computer stock control and reordering. At the same time it provides an enormous amount of information about turnover and profitability on any of the lines or goods sold within the pharmacy.

When the customer presents the goods to the assistant, the bar-code on the item is scanned at the till which, if it is an EPOS system, will send the information on the sale to the computer. The computer returns the price to the till, which then prints an itemised receipt while the computer removes the item from the stock figures. Warnings are then flagged when the stock item becomes low.

It is simple to see how useful such a tool is in any retailing environment.

References

1   The Royal Pharmaceutical Society (2002) *Guidance on Pharmacy Computer Systems. Medicines Ethics and Practice: A Guide for Pharmacists, Number 26, July 2002, Section 3.2.3, p. 102.* Royal Pharmaceutical Society of Great Britain, London.
2   British Medical Association and The Pharmaceutical Society (updated twice yearly) *British National Formulary.* BMJ Books, London.

Chapter 10

Taking stock

And that is probably what you are doing right now as you sit back and contemplate what you may have let yourself in for. Running a pharmacy, like running a dispensing practice, is no sinecure.

After your staff, your stock is the most valuable part of your pharmacy. After all, your capital is invested here.

Next time you are in town go and have a look at a few pharmacies to find out what kind of things they sell or provide for their customer-patients. You will find they broadly fit into a number of classifications:

1   ethical medicines and drugs
2   pharmacy-only medicines (P-only)
3   general sales list (GSL), otherwise known as OTC medicines
4   pharmacy-oriented products: herbals, homoeopathic drugs, nutritional, diagnostic products, maternity
5   general goods – of one sort or another as the pharmacist or owner chooses. Traditionally chemists have been involved in photographic goods.

Each of these has its specific suppliers and rewards.

Ethicals

Primarily and almost by definition a pharmacy dispenses medicines and it is this which will be concentrated on initially. Dispensing doctors may want to skip the next section but, on the other hand, as there are certain differences, they may like to read on. Non-dispensing doctors will find this to be new territory.

Generally speaking a pharmacy must be geared up to dispense any script that comes through the doors within a reasonable time, no matter what it may be for. However, the in-house pharmacy will have the great advantage of working to one group of doctors' pharmacopoeia or practice formulary and that may, or even should not, vary much from week to week or even month to month.

The advantage is that the stock carried will be of a smaller range and quantity, depending on the doctors and the pharmacist getting together and thrashing out that formulary. That does not mean simply and slavishly following the PCT's set list. Many drugs are included in that by virtue of their inexpensiveness, rather than their effectiveness, and it is, perhaps, common sense that cheap bricks do not necessarily make strong walls.

Ethicals – prescribed drugs – fall into a number of different classifications:

- branded products (parallel imports are a subdivision of branded products)
- generic products
- branded generics.

Branded products

These are generally speaking products marketed while still under patent by the company that researched, developed and manufactured them. When out of patent, other companies may develop their own copies, which may then be sold under their own brand name. Their cost to the NHS is negotiated through the Prescription Price Regulation Board (PPRB) and it is not true that the drug manufacturers fleece the government. Anybody who thinks that government cannot stand up for itself must be naïve.

Another class of branded product is the 'me-too' version of an existing drug, which varies only slightly from the first-comer, but may still be patented as a separate entity.

Parallel imports

Parallel imports are legitimate products identical to the patented drug, but possibly manufactured abroad by the same company. They are imported legally into the country without the permission of the patent holder in this country. The purpose is entirely to benefit from the difference in price between the two countries.

Generic products

Generic products are off-patent branded products produced by alternative, or even the original manufacturer under the chemical, approved name. More often than not they are produced at a cheaper cost to the NHS than the branded goods, because the makers do not have to carry out the essential research and development (R&D) work required by the originators of the drug. That, of course, has interested successive Secretaries of State, who really do believe you can build a strong house with cheap bricks.

There are arguments both ways about the use of generics and here is perhaps not the place to rehearse them all. Suffice to say that the last two Health Secretaries have even forced the price of generics down. In parallel with that, GPs are now almost being compelled to use generics whether they approve of them or not. For that reason, and for no other, the generic prescribing rate in England in 2001 was 74%. In contrast, the French and Spanish prescribe only 3% generics, the Portuguese less than 1% and in Germany 21%.

The NHS is said to have saved about £4 billion through this policy. One has to wonder what it does with the money.

The effect of continually and compulsorily reducing prices will inevitably be that the makers will seek to cut their costs. That may be done by either moving abroad or using cheaper ingredients or both. The government may at some time come to understand that, in the words of my Yorkshire countrymen, 'You don't get owt for nowt'.

Branded generics

These are neither fish nor fowl, although they tend to fall into the generic category as they are manufactured or supplied by generic companies that choose to put their own brand name on them to distinguish them from generics originating from their competitors. They often carry their own special discount arrangements for purchasers.

The PPRB and the PPA both count them as generics in their pricing and reimbursement policies.

Stocking the shelves

The purpose of this section is to give non-dispensing doctors and others some insight into the business of the pharmacy.

It now comes to the business of stocking the dispensary shelves. After all, it's no good having the most up-to-date dispensary in the country if it is not well stocked, but not overstocked. For this part of the setting-up procedure the help of the superintendent pharmacist is essential and, indeed, some may wish to leave the whole process up to them. Others may like the initial hands-on experience. It is mostly for them that the following section is written.

However, remember that the RPS Code of Ethics places full responsibility for the pharmacy on the shoulders of pharmacists. They may not welcome your help.

Overstocking may come about due to a number of causes – possibly from yielding too easily to the hordes of well-meaning reps who will pass through the doors, to stocking the wrong items – items that may not be in the practice formulary. So, I repeat, thrash that formulary out thoroughly, from time to time, with all the GPs in the health centre.

Sources of supply

There are four main sources of supply:

1   wholesalers
2   parallel importers
3   manufacturers
4   generic suppliers.

Wholesalers

There are many wholesalers – large and small – and their service is generally very good, but they may not all give the same 'deal'. It is as well to remember a fact mentioned earlier in the book, that the NHS, in its wisdom, assumes that the pharmacy will get a discount on everything it buys – almost. It is for that reason that *The Drug Tariff* has a discount deduction scale (q.v.). The appropriate percentage of the cost of the total drugs bill will be deducted by the PPA, whether or not the discount has been obtained. So, if you don't want to let the DoH dig deep into your pockets, go out and get that discount.

If you are leaving the whole thing to pharmacists, then do ensure that they keep up with the discount battle.

There is one difference between dispensing doctors and pharmacists – pharmacists have a ZD scale, which covers medicines that are used so rarely that no discount may be obtained. In these cases no discount is deducted. To their irritation, there is no such classification for dispensing doctors. Discount is deducted from the entire drugs bill.

The first step in choosing a wholesaler is to find out which ones serve your area. A list of wholesalers follows. Then ask a selection of sales managers to visit to discuss terms. Be hard-nosed – the NHS is!

There are a number of essential points that should have been satisfactorily addressed by your chosen supplier.

1   Deliveries: same day, twice daily, weekends and emergencies?
2   Stock levels: what is their 'out-of-stock' frequency rate?
3   Ordering facilities: computer or phone?
4   Stocktaking levels: are these carried out online?
5   Frequency of updates?
6   Discount offered: threshold, excluded products, extras?
7   Links to manufacturers for additional discounts?

Wholesalers include:

- AAH Pharmaceuticals Ltd (branches throughout UK); 01928 717070
- A1 Pharmaceuticals; 0207 738 7373
- BR Pharmaceuticals Ltd; 0113 256 5836
- Europharm; 0500 525381
- Freeman Pharmaceuticals; 0800 212962
- Graham Tatford; 01705 288850
- Phoenix Medical (lately Philip Harris); 0121 433 3030
- Rowlands; 01978 340100
- Sangers (NI) Ltd; 01232 401111
- Unichem; 0208 391 2323.

This list is far from comprehensive. There appears to be a wholesaler in virtually every county in the country and, of course, every pharmacy or dispensing practice is served by one or the other wholesaler. Once again, consult the *Chemist & Druggist Directory*.

Parallel importers

There are also specialist importers of parallel medicines. When ordering parallel imports from whatever source, do remember that all packaging, instructions and labelling must, by law, be in English and that includes inserts. Be sure that the supplier abides by these regulations and check all received products. Return any to the supplier that do not and do not, under any circumstances, dispense any product without English instructions and details. That would be an offence.

Parallel importers include:

- A1 Pharmaceuticals; 0500 295329
- Campdale Ltd; 01530 510520
- Chemilines Ltd; 0208 810 5001

- Europharm; 01903 845200
- Freeman Pharmaceuticals Ltd; 0800 212962
- Global Pharmaceuticals Ltd; 0208 974 2786
- Grange Pharmaceuticals; 01633 838022
- Impharm Nationwide Ltd; 01204 371155.

Manufacturers

As many dispensing doctors have found, to get the best deals here it is good policy to see as many reps as possible and to set a good relationship with them. They want to make firm contracts and are, in many cases, prepared to bargain to get one. Why not help them?

A slight aside here. It has been said that reps are not as friendly to pharmacies, so it is down to you and your superintendent pharmacist to change that.

Goods may be obtained either in bulk, with a good discount, from the reps or again from the reps, but supplied through the wholesaler. In many cases discount will be obtained from both the company and the wholesaler. It is obviously more sensible to agree that sort of deal if possible.

If ordering and buying direct from a manufacturer or their rep it is of vital importance to keep efficient records of each supplier in a separate folder. This should contain the business card of the rep, with the company and his own personal telephone numbers. Other details should be the date the deal was set up, and when it was reviewed and, if possible, the expiry date. Then should follow full details of the deal and a copy of the signed contract between the pharmacy and the company.

It then becomes the pharmacist's duty to check at regular intervals that the deal is still in operation, because companies have been known to omit to inform their customers when it no longer applies.

Dispensing practices have known for years that the rule is that it is not good policy to bulk-buy a drug to maximise profits if the product is not already being used by the doctors. It is another matter, however, if the formulary shows that the product is being used and your in-house pharmacy is in an excellent position to take advantage of that.

If, for some odd reason, that rule is ignored, then it may be that at a later date, when the cupboards are cleared, large quantities of Me-too-agem are found to be outdated and unused.

It is also good sense to check the expiry dates of delivered stock. Once again, it is not unknown for reps to deliver hundreds of packs of Me-too-agem which will outdate at the end of the month. Check, check, check! It's your company profit that will be effected.

From company through wholesaler

Technically, this is not direct purchase because a third party – the wholesaler – is involved, but many companies have been offering this system to dispensing practices, if not to pharmacies, for a considerable period of time. Your in-house pharmacy, being closely allied to the medical practice, may well be able to obtain similar deals to dispensing doctors.

Company discount is based on the usage of their product. Your invoices or the stock usage figures, obtained with your written consent, from your wholesaler suffices as evidence of that.

At least one company is now using a wholesaler as the preferred agent for the sales of its products and the discount is often across the board for almost its whole range of products.

Other firms may request permission for a company rep to seek your sensitive purchase information from your wholesaler before giving discount. If agreeing to this, be sure to review the arrangement from time to time and that rather than becoming permanent, it does lapse with the end of any contract you may sign. Your wholesaler will be able to remind you to whom you have given this permission.

The benefit of these arrangements are that they are based on pharmaceuticals that are already being used by the practice, and therefore by the pharmacy, and extra capital is not required. Another benefit is that the bonus obtained from the company is usually in addition to the wholesaler discount. It may also be boosted by the rep, by discount in kind, on his routine visit to the pharmacy.

Generic suppliers
As always, the list that follows is not comprehensive. More suppliers may be found by consulting the advertisers and listings in reputable pharmaceutical magazines.

When using the list it would be as well to bear in mind that where the wholesaler (see above) may well be able to supply a comprehensive list of generic medicines, many of the generic suppliers, otherwise known as 'short-line' suppliers, listed below will have only a limited list. However, the benefit is that they may well be offered at a large discount. That is the good side – the bad side is that cheap is not necessarily good. So, in a word, beware – in some cases.

A final comment. It is possible to find some supplier-manufacturers which supply only single, difficult-to-obtain drugs. *The Chemist & Druggist Directory*[1] may be helpful in searching them out.

The inclusion of any company in this list is no guarantee in any way.

- APS Berk Generics; 0800 590502
- Global Pharmaceuticals Ltd; 0208 974 2786
- Baker Norton Ltd; 01635 563000
- Doncaster Pharmaceuticals Ltd; 01302 886031
- Shire Pharmaceuticals Ltd; 01264 333455.

Specials
At some time or other the doctors will prescribe medications that may only be made under a *specials* manufacturing licence. These items may be difficult to supply and it will almost never be possible to do so on the same day.

A 'specials' supplier is: The Specials Laboratory; 0800 028 4925.

The retail side

A good pharmacy will have found its own special niche market, maybe from one of the areas mentioned below.

When deciding what to sell it is sensible to have a few ground rules.

1   Stock the right goods at the right price.
2   Try to specialise in a particular area of product.

3   Try to find out what your customers like and want.
4   Do not stock slow-selling goods – they ruin the profit margins.
5   Do not bulk purchase unless EPOS (q.v.) gives evidence of rapid sales.
6   Do not stock more than two days' supply – if deliveries are good.
7   Keep a good range of GSL, P and healthcare items.
8   Check with the medical practice what they may recommend to patients.
9   Ensure the staff are friendly and the premises attractive.
10   Use retail psychology to display your stock.

Pharmacy-oriented products

Included among these are:

- homoeopathic medicines
- herbals
- nutrients
- baby foods
- bladder products
- feminine products
- eyecare
- contraceptive supplies.

Homoeopathic medicines

One of the better established alternative medical treatments, homoeopathy, was introduced some 200 years ago by Samuel Hahman, a German pharmacist. Homoeopathic medicines are said to cure without toxicity, interactions or side effects.

From the pharmacy point of view, homoeopathy is profitable, having profit margins of 40%–50% and private consultations with a trained homoeopathist can bring in over £50 an hour.

There are specialist suppliers of these medicines:

- Ainsworth (London) Ltd; 0207 935 5330
- Bioforce (UK) Ltd; 01294 277344
- MB Grant Ltd; 0114 264 4455
- A Nelson & Co Ltd; 0208 780 4200
- Weleda (UK) Ltd; 0115 944 8200.

Herbals

Doctors and pharmacists should be constantly aware of possible interactions between herbal medicines and ethical medicines. It certainly cannot be said that just because it is herbal and sold OTC, it is completely safe. After all, digoxin is derived from that well-known plant the foxglove and nobody in their right senses would claim that it is safe in all circumstances.

Despite this an increasing number of people are put off ethical medicines by all the potential side-effects described on the mandatory pack inserts, and are rushing towards herbals. They are sold at large prices and large profits and so long as the pharmacy has a professional attitude towards them then they may be sold.

Some may say that selling them in a pharmacy is a better place than elsewhere. Obviously some would disagree with that. In any case, customers will ask about them. An excellent reference book is *Herbal Medicines: a guide for healthcare professionals*[2] and a copy should be on every pharmacy, if not every doctor's, bookshelf. It is available on a CD-ROM.

As with ethical pharmaceuticals, selling herbals without a knowledge of what is being sold is not professional. If they are to be stocked then ensure that the pharmacist and the counter assistant have a working knowledge or, at the very least, are prepared to look up unknown queries.

The first question anybody who sells herbal preparations and remedies should ask the customer is, 'Are you on any other medications?', and then go on to check them out against the requested herbal.

There are many suppliers of herbal remedies of which the following are but a few:

- Bioforce (UK) Ltd; 01294 277344
- Peter Black Healthcare Ltd; 01283 228300
- Ferrosan Healthcare Ltd; 01932 337700
- Health Imports Ltd; 01274 488511
- Jessup Marketing; 01932 854825
- GR Lane Health Products Ltd; 01452 524012
- Linpharma Herbal Products; 01506 848 649
- Moducare; 01782 567100
- Natra Health; 01753 864455
- Potters Herbal Supplies Ltd; 01942 234761.

Nutrients

Pharmacies are often the first port of call for advice on diets and nutrients, so pharmacists and their staff should be well briefed on this wide-ranging subject and know when it is right to intervene. In the National Service Framework (NSF) for the elderly, the NHS has highlighted nutrition as a problem to be addressed for this group.

Nutritional supplements may well be especially indicated in the debilitated, anorexic or post-operative elderly. Some are available on prescription; others are sold OTC as drinks, chocolate bars or pills.

Own branding

Nutrients generate good profitability for the pharmacy and that profitability may be increased by putting your own pharmacy name on the label – own branding. This is said to tell the customer that your pharmacy has faith in what it is selling.

Own-brand labels should only carry the details of your pharmacy and none of your suppliers.

As with any pharmacy-oriented product your staff should not offer advice to customers if they are not sure what they are talking about. The WHICH? report[3] of February 2004 showed only too well how many pharmacies and their staff were prepared to give the wrong advice rather than find out what the good advice should be. That is not good enough. Your pharmacy is a part of the healthcare centre and as such its staff must be well informed.

The following is a relatively short list of suppliers of nutrient products. There are many more, some dealing in only a very short range of preparations.

- Bellwether Nutrition (will 'own-brand'); 01639 813555
- BR Pharmaceuticals; 0113 256 5836
- Chemist Brokers; 01705 222500
- Efamol Ltd; 01483 304441
- Fresenius; 01928 579444
- Lagap Pharmaceuticals Ltd; 01420 478301
- Natures Own Ltd; 01684 310022
- Nutricia Life; 08457 623686: www.nutriplus.co.uk
- Vitabiotics Ltd; 0208 963 0999.

Baby foods

Here, too, pharmacies are often the first call for advice – after the visiting midwife has stopped calling. Many new mothers prefer not to disturb the ever-willing health visitor over what some see as a trivial matter. Your in-house pharmacy will, of course, be able to take advantage of your attached health visitor's advice by selling the very products she recommends.

As with everything else be sure that the staff are familiar with the concept of both breast- and bottle-feeding and that their advice will be good advice.

Supplement that advice with informative leaflets and with a competitively priced range of baby products. That includes bottles, teats, sterilising equipment and various feeds and foods, and show it in an attractive way. By doing this your pharmacy will gain the new mother's trust – and custom. It should not be forgotten that young mothers spend, on average, 30% more than other customers. Oh, and don't forget those nappies!

This list of suppliers is necessarily incomplete in an enormous market.

Babycare
- Avent; 0800 289064: www.avent.com
- Galpharm International Ltd; 01226 779911
- Johnson & Johnson Ltd; 01628 822222
- J Pickles; 01423 867314.

Baby feeding
- Babytec Ltd; 01258 459554
- Lewis Woolf Griptight Ltd; 01386 553386
- Sterifeed – Brandbeat Ltd; 01823 673062.

Baby foods
- HJ Heinz; 0208 573 7757
- Mead Johnson; 0208 754 3764
- SMA Nutrition Ltd; 01628 660633.

Nappies
- Kimberley-Clark Ltd; 01622 616000
- Premier Disposables Ltd; 01273 477370
- Procter & Gamble; 0191 279 2000.

Bladder products

Apart from enuresis in youngsters most of this market is directed towards the middle-aged and elderly of both sexes.

Bed wetting
Astoundingly, enuresis is said to be a problem at some time for one in six children between the ages of five and 16. After visiting the doctor or the health visitor the patient will sooner or later turn up at the pharmacy for supplies and advice. It is a very socially disruptive and even destructive condition. Many children refuse to stay away from home when all the rest of their friends will enjoy nights away at each others' homes. Some will not even go on holiday, fearing the assumed disgrace of a nightly wet bed.

The pharmacy is in an ideal position to provide support.

- Helplines for bed-wetting:

  – bed-wetting helpline; 0800 085 8189
  – PromoCon; 0161 834 2001

- Supplies:

  – Kimberley-Clark; 0800 085 8189.

Adult incontinence
The NHS can, but does not always, provide through *The Drug Tariff* a wide range of incontinence products and pads. In practice, however, many patients will turn to other suppliers and the chief of these will be the pharmacy. No doubt advice will be given by the practice or district nurse and products may be purchased at the in-house pharmacy.

The figures show that over six million people in this country suffer with bladder weakness of one degree or another – a sizeable market by any standards, considering that it is a chronic problem for which, in many cases, there is no treatment – only care.

Once again the pharmacist and staff must be well up to date on what is a very distressing problem to virtually all sufferers. It is here where the confidential area will be in great demand for the pharmacist to run through all the options of treatment and protective products. It should not be forgotten that there are treatments and also that incontinence may mask a more serious condition. Staff should have a low threshold for referring the customer to the doctors for diagnostic help.

Many customers may be too embarrassed to enquire about products and prefer to quickly choose an item from the display. The pharmacy can help this by displaying a comprehensive – but not too comprehensive – range of products, arranged in order of absorbancy. A description of each could be shown on the shelf front to aid choice.

An additional aid would be a tactful display of self-help leaflets describing the condition and what can be done about it. Suppliers include:

- Comforta Healthcare Ltd; 01905 356524
- Femcare Ltd; 0115 978 6322
- Hygicare Ltd 01978 363300
- Maersk Medical Ltd; 01527 64222
- Richardsons; 0116 273 6571
- SCA Hygiene Products Ltd; 01582 677400
- Tena; 0870 333 0874.

Feminine products

It is pretty safe to say that most women will have made their minds up about which sanitary protection product to use. A comprehensive range of products is essential, arranged discretely, according to whether they are pads, towels or tampons. It would be helpful if most displays could be at eye-level, as with incontinence products. Once again, leaflets may well be useful, particularly for young girls embarking on this stage of their lives. Suppliers include:

- Cannon Hygiene Ltd; 01524 60894
- Johnson & Johnson Ltd; 01628 822222
- Kimberley-Clark Ltd; 01622 616000
- Ontex Ltd; 01536 269744.

In addition to these feminine products there are a number of GSL products available, which could be displayed alongside.

Eyecare

There is some controversy as to whether this is an appropriate subject for pharmacy sales except, possibly, in the larger branches of, for instance, Boots. Many opticians are unhappy with pharmacies that sell corrective spectacles without carrying out an eye test of any kind.

As the pharmacy under discussion here is part of a 'one-stop' primary care centre, which will have its own optician, it is perhaps not appropriate for it to sell anything other than, for instance, contact lens sterilising solutions. On the other hand, the pharmacist could take advantage of the proximity of the optician to decide which other products may be retailed.

Suppliers of contact lens accessories include:

- Aspect Vision Care; 01442 876488
- Bausch & Lomb UK Ltd; 0208 781 2986
- CIBA Vision Ltd; 01489 785399.

Contraceptive supplies

Although there are slot machines in many public toilets and barbers still occasionally sell condoms, the main outlets are still the pharmacy or petrol station.

They should be on open display at the cash counter where they may be readily chosen. Suppliers include:

- Chemist Brokers; 01705 222500
- FP Sales Ltd; 01865 749333
- LRC Products Ltd; 01992 451111
- London International Group Ltd; 0207 489 1977
- WJ Rendall Ltd; 01462 432596
- Safex Supplies Ltd; 01782 723399.

Pregnancy test kits
Many years ago most HAs, as they then were, withdrew funding for pregnancy testing. Some surgeries continued to help their patients out at some cost to themselves. It is possible that very few of these beneficent GPs remain and that more and more pregnancy tests will be obtained OTC from pharmacies.

Pharmacy staff are in the right place to be able to offer a comprehensive help service. Suppliers include:

- ARC Pharmacare Ltd; 01204 362236
- BR Pharmaceuticals; 0113 256 5836
- Kent Pharmaceuticals Ltd; 01233 638614
- Organon Teknika Ltd; 01223 423650
- Unipath Ltd; 01234 835 000.

Summary

It is very possible that readers will be able to add other pharmacy-oriented items to the above list, but the ones mentioned will be sufficient to get the pharmacy on its feet and keep customers loyal.

Keen readers will have noticed that several of the products may be obtained from one or more of the comprehensive wholesalers listed earlier. It is certainly worth looking at their prices, but individual suppliers should not be neglected. However, the more suppliers used the greater the administrative work for the pharmacist in keeping up with orders. The counter staff should be trained to help by keeping a record of all sales and shortages as they occur. In the more modern pharmacy, such as yours, of course, this may well be carried out by the EPOS computer system.

General retail goods

There are two constraints on retailing a larger selection of goods. The first is the lack of an inclination to do so and the second is space. To those could be added a third constraint, which is the appropriateness of the item for sale in a pharmacy. It would not do for pharmacies to sell tobacco and related products, for instance. In any case, the RPS would have something to say to the pharmacist who did sell cigarettes.

Hair care, cosmetics, male care, toiletries all come to mind here as items that many people would expect to find in a pharmacy of moderate size. No doubt you or your pharmacist will be able to add to that not very comprehensive list.

So far as profit is concerned, however, in comparison with the list of pharmacy-related products, such retail items will not add very much. However, what may do so is photographic developing and printing, now that this is completely automated. On the other hand, is that a band wagon to jump on now that so many digital cameras are being sold? Your guess is as good as mine. But if you do decide to jump, then there are commercial digital camera developing units available.

As this is a specialist subject then whoever looks after it should take the trouble to learn the subject well. If customer photos do not 'come out' well, then word will soon spread. Suppliers of photographic equipment include:

* Fujifilm; 01234 217724: www.fujifilm.co.uk
* Gretag; 0870 870 8321
* Mitsubishi Electric Europe; 01707 278684: www.mitsubishi.co.uk/evs.

References

1 *Chemist & Druggist Directory* (published annually by CMP Data & Information, Tonbridge).
2 Barnes J, Anderson LA and Phillipson JD (2002) *Herbal Medicines: a guide for healthcare professionals* (2e). Pharmaceutical Press, London.
3 *WHICH? Pharmacy* (February 2004) WHICH?, London.

Chapter 11

Any other matters

This is a chapter of items which do not fit easily into any of the earlier chapters. Included are:

- care of the disabled
- clinical governance in pharmacy
- dump schemes
- medicines management in pharmacy
- minor ailments and pharmacy
- NHS Direct and pharmacy
- non-prescription medicine monitoring
- out-of-hours care
- PCTs and pharmacy
- risk management
- use of the confidential area.

Care of the disabled

The Disability Discrimination Act (DDA) (q.v.) describes disablement as: 'a physical or mental impairment which has a substantial and long-term effect on (the disabled person's) ability to carry out his normal day-to-day activities'. Somewhat astoundingly, almost one-sixth of the adult population of this country fits into that classification. Small wonder that their special needs are being seriously catered for. The disabilities include:

- hearing impairment
- visual impairment
- speech impairment
- incontinence
- dementia
- mobility problems.

All these people must be able to use the services of the pharmacy in the same way as would the unimpaired customer.

Hearing, visual and speech impairment

The first maxim for any worker consulted by an impaired person is to remember that long running Radio 4 programme for the disabled, 'Does he take sugar?' This quite rightly and vigorously drew attention to the plain, unvarnished fact that the disabled person is, indeed, a person in his own right. Always address him directly and not his helpers, unless advised otherwise.

The hearing impaired may already have hearing aids, but if there is a difficulty then simply writing notes or providing leaflets may well be sufficient.

The visually impaired could be helped by large, bold print or by an assistant who is prepared to interpret the writing on labels or read leaflets.

The speech impaired may be provided with writing materials.

Wheelchair users

They, of course, need to be able to gain entry to the pharmacy and, as mentioned earlier, this may be by a ramp – permanent or moveable – or with the help of an assistant prepared to manoeuvre the chair over any steps. In addition, the door should be wide enough to permit entry as should any checkout counter and there must be no impassable obstructions within the shop. The Regulation demanding that reasonable measures be provided for the access of the disabled came into force on 1 October 2004.

The NPA is a mine of information and help, and will be prepared to advise and provide the names and addresses of the providers of suitable materials or devices.

Clinical governance in pharmacy

There is a DoH definition of clinical governance:

> The framework through which NHS organisations are accountable for continuously improving the quality of their services and safeguarding high standards of care by creating an environment in which excellence in clinical care can flourish.

The RPS has issued national guidance to pharmacies, which must be followed. It consists of:

* maintaining the quality of clinical care by means of clear lines of responsibility
* the adoption of a quality improvement programme, to include:
  – audit
  – continuing professional development (CPD)
  – effective monitoring of clinical activities
  – evidence-based practice.
* a risk management policy (q.v. in this chapter)
* the recognition and correction of inadequate performance.

Audit

In clinical discussions the term 'audit' means observing what is happening and has occurred and learning from it.

Continuing professional development

All professionals must keep themselves up to date and in a proper position to carry out their duties by a programme of continuous learning.

Effective monitoring of clinical practice

Without this, audit is impossible.

Evidence-based practice

Evidence-based practice consists of only carrying out tasks that have been proven to be effective. If there's no proof it works, don't do it sounds very dogmatic, but that is the implication. It is the antithesis of innovation.

All these points are involved in clinical governance and it is to this end that the PCO has appointed a pharmacy clinical governance facilitator with the help of the LPC. There will also be a community pharmacist on the PCT Board, if they can find one who has time to serve.

The facilitator should form links with outside pharmacy groups such as the NPA, the RPSGB and the LPC in order to find how they can contribute to the programme of governance. The NPA has developed a three-year development plan for England and Wales, which has been agreed by the clinical governance facilitator and local pharmacists.

Following on from all this the RPS will expect that written standard operating procedures (SOPs) for dispensing are in place in all pharmacies by 1 January 2005.

Be sure that your new pharmacy is in a position to fulfil all the new strictures of clinical governance. They include staff and pharmacist training, patient access, as mentioned earlier and even policies to be carried out when drugs are recalled by the manufacturers.

At present, participation in clinical governance may be voluntary, but there are plans for the future.

The PCO is asked by the Healthcare Commission to provide such information as will permit the Commission to consider the service provided by community pharmacies under the following heads:

- patient and public involvement
- managing risks
- clinical audit
- the use of clinical information
- staffing and staff management
- education, training and CPD
- clinical effectiveness.

All these may be enshrined in the new pharmacy contract, so it would be as well for your superintendent pharmacist to be in a position where all the pharmacy staff can comply. The LPC will be able to give up-to-the-minute help and advice.

DUMP schemes

It is an unfortunate fact of life that for many reasons patients do not always use all the medicines they order and, from time to time, pharmacies need to have a DUMP campaign to have them returned out of harms way.

Prescription-only medicines are subject to control under the Special Waste Regulations and when returned to pharmacies must be disposed of according to those Regulations. However, the Regulations do not apply to the householder who disposes of them at home. The causes for superfluous medicines being in patients' homes include:

- side effects and consequent non-compliance with medication
- over-ordering of 'repeats' – common among the elderly
- change of medicine regime either by the GP or the hospital doctors
- the death of the patient.

An alert pharmacist, whose dispensary is consistently used by the patient, will be in a good position to monitor individual patients' repeat medicines and, hopefully, prevent the accumulation of vast quantities of expensive and dangerous medications in peoples' homes. The in-house pharmacy is ideally placed in this respect.

The DUMP campaign could be an annual, well-publicised event. Local newspapers may be happy to place the story as a news item and send a photographer round at the end of the campaign period to photograph the result.

The PCO should be involved as it may be about to run an area scheme, but in any case it could help with the disposal of the returned drugs. It will also give advice about their temporary storage to prevent them falling into the wrong hands. If the PCO is unable to help then the usual waste disposal firms should be consulted (see below).

The pharmacy should provide a suitable container for the collection of these drugs until they are collected by a registered or licensed waste disposal firm. The object is to make the drugs unusable and that may be done by shelling out pills from calendar packs before dropping them in a concentrated mixture of, for example, detergent and liquid polish.

Pharmacies do not need a licence for the collection, although any pharmacist who collects waste medications in the course of their business will need to be registered. Details may be obtained from the Environment Agency on 08459 333 111.

Disposal services include:

- DOOP Services; 01491 612267
- Pharma Waste Ltd; 01903 820574.

DOOP offer CD waste disposal kits for pharmacies and dispensing practices.

Medicines management in pharmacy

The approved definition of medicines management is: 'to optimise prescribing, health outcomes and patient experiences where medicines are involved'. Or, in short, helping people to get the most from their medicines.

All PCTs should have had medicines management schemes in place by April 2004 and at the time of writing it is not known whether such schemes will become part of the pharmacist's New Contract.

The Medicines Management Services (MMS) programme is based in Liverpool and collaborates with PCTs which, themselves, have a project team of a dozen people. Commonly they are community pharmacists, PCT prescribing advisers and, possibly, GP representatives. Their purpose is to identify good and bad practice and to pass on the knowledge gained from doing that.

The teams have looked at care homes and how visits from community pharmacists could help patients and staff understand and administer drugs better. They have also studied repeat prescribing in an attempt to identify if and why patients ask for medicines they don't need and whether they are taking the ones they are given.

Following these studies, in some parts of the country it has been seen that compliance has increased and prescribing or presentation of repeats has been improved by a reduction in the number of items requested. There has been some anxiety among community pharmacists as to whether this will affect their income.

All this has been carried out by the project teams liaising with GPs, patient organisations, health visitors, nurses and social workers.

In nine areas of the UK the project teams have focused on particular disease entities, cardiovascular disease being one. Large numbers of patients with this condition in these areas were randomly chosen and split into two groups. Half were used as controls and received standard pharmacy treatment, while the others were subject to an intervention project. The intervention was designed to maximise health gain for the patient together with cost-efficient prescribing for the NHS, improving cooperation between pharmacists and other professionals, and making the most of the pharmacist's skills. Participating pharmacists are paid for their time. The trial is being evaluated by the Universities of Aberdeen, Keele and Nottingham.

Patients are said to have reacted positively to the trials and the response of other professionals is being evaluated as the trial proceeds.

This project is specifically designed for a community pharmacy setting and seeks to make the most out of the accessibility of the community pharmacists and their knowledge of the patient. The robust nature of the trial is intended to provide evidence of the value of the pharmacist's place in the primary care team.

It may or may not detract from the project, but random high-street chemists and pharmacies were not used as participants. Instead, to quote the PSNC document on the project:[1]

> There was a thorough training programme for all those involved in the project and this was organised and delivered by the Centre for Pharmacy Postgraduate Education.

Much will be made, politically, of the outcome of the trial, but whether that will relate to anywhere other than these trained centres of excellence is debatable. Will the average high-street pharmacist be able to deliver the same results without special training?

So far as your in-house pharmacy is concerned, it is vitally important that, as a medically owned pharmacy, it delivers care to the highest possible standard. The opportunity for close collaboration with the medical practice is greater than at most high-street chemists and there will be many eyes upon the service it provides. For that reason you may wish to seek to involve it in medicine management schemes.

Minor ailments and pharmacy

Much has been written about this topic, mostly by pharmacists seeking an alternative role to dispensing, which if modern safeguards are adopted does, nowadays, consist largely of sticking a label on a box.

Pharmacists are keen to reduce the GP's workload in this way but, oddly, not so keen when the dispensing GP attempts to lessen the pharmacist's workload. This keenness is reflected in *The NHS Plan*[2], which supports pharmacy's aspirations as an alleged step in its own demands for the 24–48-hour access target for patients visiting GP surgeries.

Interestingly, considering that the exercise is designed, we are told, to reduce GP workload, a survey in Sefton in 2001[3] showed no impact whatsoever on total GP workload when the scheme was adopted there.

Other trials have been undertaken elsewhere, where the chemist is paid a £300 retainer and medicines are free to patients, but reimbursed to the chemist at cost price.

If your pharmacy is to take part in such a scheme – or simply just treat minor ailments as they arrive – then it is vital that the staff know which conditions they may offer remedies for and which not. They should also be trained in minor ailments and be aware when to refer firstly to the pharmacist and secondly to the doctors. The training should be continuous. The free magazine *Training Matters*[4] from the Communications International Group provides an excellent source of continuous learning for pharmacy staff. There is also an excellent book on the subject: *OTC Medications: symptoms and treatments of common illnesses.*[5]

It is becoming obvious that in the near future pharmacists will be allowed their own prescribing list, derived from the previously POM-only list. Unless your pharmacist is well-trained, possibly by the health centre doctors, the possibility for the occasional disaster may well present itself.

Whenever the pharmacist or staff treat patients under official schemes a record must be made of that treatment, including full details of the suspected condition, date and the treatment given. However, when patients simply buy OTC preparations to self-medicate, no record is needed.

Not only will such records improve patient safety, but they will also provide a valuable audit tool for research purposes at a later date.

One leading pharmacy politician, Mr S Dajani, claims that the benefits outweigh the risk and that there are financial savings to the NHS. There is, he says, one major remaining challenge – funding. There is no universal fee structure, he complains.

Many doctors wonder whether releasing more prescription-only drugs onto the pharmacy list is wise until all pharmacists, not just some, are fully trained in the diagnostic skills that take GPs five or six undergraduate years, plus several postgraduate years, to acquire.

Until then the concept remains a politically motivated scheme being adopted by a government faced with a long-term shortage of doctors, which it is failing to address effectively.

In short, by all means have your pharmacy treat *minor ailments* suitable for self-medication, but ensure that the pharmacist is fully trained and prepared to take full and personal responsibility for doing so. This might be mentioned at the pharmacist's interview.

NHS Direct and pharmacy

Recent research has revealed that 40% of NHS Direct enquiries involved medicines in one way or another. That being so, it was essential that the nurses running the call service had access to pharmaceutical advice, either directly or online. It was also essential that they had some training in pharmacy and that the organisation had pharmacy input from the start. All this has been achieved.

The nurses now understand when to refer callers to pharmacy and when to refer to other primary care services, mainly GPs or hospital A&E departments. They should have been provided with the on-call, out-of-hours arrangements for pharmacies in the caller's area.

For their part, community pharmacists should feed back their experiences to NHS Direct call centres and be prepared, as high-street pharmacists, to help train nurses for the centres.

The future may hold massive developments for patients. NHS Direct nurses may be able to order medicines for the patient directly to the pharmacy of their choice. Your pharmacy may wish to take advantage of this when it comes about.

The system sounds perfect, but there must be safeguards. For instance, the caller must be able to identify themselves in some way, as the patient, in order to prevent the fraudulent and dangerous supply of drugs. In addition, both the doctor and the pharmacist must be informed immediately of, or preferably before, the supply of any prescription medication, because this is coming perilously close to indirect, distant-nurse prescribing with all the dangers inherent in such a scheme. The question of practicality arises here. Another question is how many NHS Direct nurses will be prepared to take the responsibility for their action when they fully understand what may be asked of them?

To summarise, your pharmacy may be involved in the NHS Direct system in a number of ways.

1   It may be contacted for help and advice by NHS Direct.
2   It may be asked to dispense for unknown patients by e-pharmacy.
3   The pharmacist may be involved in nurse training for NHS Direct.
4   The pharmacist may be involved out of hours.
5   It should participate in feedback with NHS Direct.
6   The pharmacist may be asked to deliver medicines to patients.
7   The pharmacist may be asked to communicate with GPs.

The similar but far from identical scheme in Scotland is called NHS-24. Scots pharmacists are asked to look out for NHS-24 mailings and to log onto the website.

Non-prescription medicine monitoring

More and more medicines are being deregulated from POM to P-only or even to GSL and the risk of any of these self-purchased medicines adversely interreacting with prescribed medicines is also greatly increased. One very good reason why rural dispensing practices should be permitted to sell and record the sales of such medications is that such sales will be automatically checked with the patient's medication records by the dispensary computer system.

The pharmacy, particularly the primary care centre pharmacy, is in a very good position to monitor the purchase and usage of these drugs. But no pharmacy should permit its staff to sell P-only medicines without a drug history, allergies and current medication, being taken first. Many of the drugs currently released as being safe for general use can, in certain circumstances, kill.

Ibuprofen, for instance, may precipitate a catastrophic gastrointestinal haemorrhage or a fatal asthmatic attack. If the question is raised at an inquest, your pharmacy could be held to be negligent if no history is taken.

A history of all such purchases could be made in the PMR and this could be passed on to the medical practice. Interestingly, recent research by Porteous et al.[6] showed that pharmacists would be willing to do that if they were appropriately remunerated; GPs thought it would be helpful if pharmacists did relay such information, but fewer than half of patients would agree to it.

The Yellow Card System for reporting the adverse effects of drugs applies to GSL medicines just as it does to POMs and P medicines and the more pharmacists who make such reports the safer the list of pharmacy sales medicines will be.

Out-of-hours care

It has long been the politician's vote-catching dream that the NHS as an entirety would be 'open all hours'. Whether this availability-at-all-costs culture is good for anybody is questionable. However, they said it and we, as healthcare providers, appear to have to get on with it. So do pharmacies and their staff.

A better out-of-hours service was promised as long ago as 2002 in *The NHS Modernisation Plan*. It was repeated in *Pharmacy in the Future*,[7] which expected pharmacies to work closely with NHS Direct. It attempted to ensure that patients who needed common medicines could get them whenever they wanted them at the time of consultation and that urgent drugs were dispensed in a well-coordinated fashion.

NHS nurses are trained to only refer patients who need an urgent face-to-face consultation out of hours to the appropriate provider. This is not as easy as it may appear, because nurses, at a distance from the patient and their problem, are understandably reluctant to take responsibility for potential mishaps and the headlines they would bring with them.

There is a DoH formulary for out-of-hours medicines and these are to be dispensed in full courses by the person who sees the patient at the time of the consultation. There is not to be any funding for a national pharmacy out-of-hours scheme.

This implies that medicines will be provided from places other than pharmacies – probably by doctors. Pharmacy, ever primarily conscious of its back, sees this as a threat. If GPs can provide full courses out of hours, they ask, what is to stop them doing so in hours? Perish the thought that patients would benefit in some way by being provided with their medicines by the professional who understands their case and who has had some pharmaceutical training.

Far better, they continue, for the patient to see a properly remunerated pharmacist out of hours. In effect the NPA is saying that your pharmacist should be paid twice – once for seeing the patient and again for supplying the medicine. As a pharmacy owner you may agree.

At present, before the implementation of the new pharmacy contract, individual pharmacies may contract with their PCO to provide an out-of-hours service or, alternatively, may choose to be open without contracting to do so.

It is between you and the pharmacist what you decide to do, bearing in mind the costs involved. The new contract may shed more light on all this. Whatever is decided, the pharmacy should notify NHS Direct, the PCO and the local press of the decision. It should also be included in its practice leaflet.

PCTs and pharmacy

It is said that PCTs were formed with the intention of putting the public and local clinicians at the forefront of local healthcare provision. The clinicians would be closely involved so they could input their professional expertise into the clinical needs of the service while the lay members of the PCT injected the patient's position into the proceedings.

Very early on, the professionals who practice in the high-street – opticians and chemists – were seen to be an underused NHS resource. Pharmacists are felt to be in an ideal position to provide health promotion and health improvement propaganda.

They are also seen by the PCT to have a role, as mentioned above, in medicine management and in cutting down a possible source of NHS waste through managing, at practice level, the drugs budget. Some doctors see this as being heavy-handed when the PCT transmits strongly worded, no-nonsense apparent diktats informing them what they must prescribe in the interest of the NHS. Neither PCT managers nor PCT pharmacy advisers are in the position to know what the patient actually needs at the time, and to doctors, that is what counts above everything else.

All this apart, the pharmacist must still see the PCT as being 'Head Office', from which both his pay and his working directives emanate. It would be as well if there were good relations between them, even as the new contract passes more and more tasks from other health providers onto their backs, with or without extra remuneration.

Risk management

No health professional ever passes a day at work without there being some risk to themselves or their patients. It may be trivial, it may be major, but that risk is there. Risk management is all about identifying those risks and doing whatever is possible to eliminate them.

The risks in pharmacy are all too plain to see – especially for a dispensing doctor. The right medicine must go to the right patient at the right strength and over the right period of time – and it must not interact adversely with current medications.

But there are other, non-clinical risks for the pharmacist, mostly relating to the business:

- financial risks of the business
- purchasing stock that will sell
- looking after the staff according to all the laws and regulations
- all the Health & Safety issues involving customers, patients and staff.

Of prime concern is the dispensing process, because this is where more people are potentially at risk when the large number of dispensed items that pass through the dispensary every day are taken into account.

The pharmacy must have a dispensing protocol or standard operative procedure (SOP), and this must involve the employment of modern IT technology and the checking of each dispensed item by the pharmacist before it is released to the patient. In drawing up this protocol the whole process should be analysed to determine where mistakes are most likely to be made so that prevention may come into action.

There is an effective dispensing protocol for dispensing practices in *The Complete Dispenser* by David Roberts.[8] It will require little modification for use in a pharmacy dispensary.

Medication errors may occur as a consequence of:

- poor prescribing
- wrong dispensing
- bad administration.

Having identified these it should be possible to eliminate the first two and, with efficient legible labelling and instructions, reduce the risk of the last.

Another way of avoiding risks is by making others aware of your own mistakes and it is now essential that primary care contractors, doctors and chemists, report their errors to the National Patient Safety Agency (NPSA).

Having identified the risk and passed that knowledge on to the staff, it remains to find a risk-avoidance technique. Maybe that will be a SOP, as used throughout the profession. SOPs identify the risk, give examples and provide avoidance measures.

From 1 January 2005 all pharmacies will be required by the RPS to have in place, and to operate, a dispensing SOP.

But dispensing is not the only risky part of pharmacy. The pharmacy as a whole should be examined for potential risks of harm to customers. They may fall or may come to harm as displays come crashing on their heads. Then there are the little boys who get up to endless mischief – or you should assume they do – and come to some harm with one of your many dangerous products or devices.

Any self-respecting pharmacy designer should be capable of building in risk management. It is then down to the properly briefed staff to maintain those standards.

And don't forget, the staff are people, too, and their rest quarters, for instance, will need to be considered. Is that bank of lockers secured properly?

Finally, it may concentrate the mind for you and your pharmacist to recall that we now live in a very litigious society, inhabited by hoards of no-win no-fee solicitors just aching to take the company to court. Always, but always keep alert to potential hazards within the shop.

Use of the confidential area

The confidential area could have many uses and should be carefully and tastefully fitted out as suggested earlier. The object is to make the customer feel relaxed and at ease so that they will be able to discuss what may be very personal and sensitive problems without any fear of being overheard or, even, overlooked.

Confidential counselling

This could include pregnancy testing, sex counselling and contraception. Some customers may feel happier discussing even relatively minor problems such as constipation and the best laxative to use, with the pharmacist in this area.

Near-patient testing

A whole batch of these tests has already been mentioned in Chapter 8. It should, however, be the maxim of the pharmacy that no test will be offered or carried out without there being available proper and rapid medical counselling by a doctor in the case of an adverse result. The in-house pharmacy is in a better position by far to ensure this than any high-street chemist. On the other hand, many physicians would say that there is no place for ad hoc pharmacy testing of potentially lethal or otherwise serious conditions. Far better that the anxious customer be referred to the doctor for investigation and advice.

The medical partners will be able to advise which diagnostic tests are appropriate for provision in their pharmacy.

Travel advice

The pharmacy will be in an excellent position to help customers with advice and to sell essential travel items, following a consultation here or with the practice nurse. A pharmacist who is current with this advice will be able to help the patient choose the correct malaria prophylaxis, insecticides, insect repellents and even mosquito nets.

To be in the best position to advise customers the pharmacist should be frequently briefed by the medical practitioners.

Before advising the customer, the pharmacist should take a personal medical history together with current medications, then the details of the proposed foreign travel and the style of travel – hotel, backpacking, cruising or whatever. The advice should match the trip and the country involved.

There is plenty of advice online for the pharmacist to pass on to the customer and it will mostly generate income for the pharmacy.

Allergies

Allergy testing is a specialised procedure and there are very few centres in the country able to carry out a full diagnostic allergy test. Where the pharmacy comes in is in the provision of a treatment for the presumed allergy, the commonest of which is hay fever. The pharmacist may be able to help in the differential clinical diagnosis between perennial rhinitis, caused by house dust mites, and hay fever. The pharmacist will also be able to refer customers to the health centre doctors.

Recent figures have shown that the so-called allergy market is worth £64 million a year and grows by 17% each year, mostly in hay-fever treatments. Ever since many antihistamines became deregulated from POMs to P-only medicines there has been a rapid uptake in self-medication. A very important fact is that the medications actually work if the diagnosis is correct.

Anti-smoking advice

Once again, the patient pharmacist is in a good position to be able to help those customers who are determined to stop smoking. Advice and a number of medications that work can be provided. They work, though, only if the customer is determined to stop and has the willpower to do so.

It is not good enough just to send the customer away with a leaflet, a help line and a pack of chewing gum. That neither helps the patient nor generates future custom. The customer should be invited back on a number of occasions to boost his morale and show that somebody is interested in helping him.

The NHS does not yet pay the pharmacist a fee for this service, but a leading pharmacy politician has estimated that the profit on one of the nicotine replacement preparations should be sufficient recompense.

Alternative medicine counselling

The go-ahead pharmacy may be able to attract regular sessions from one or more alternative medicine counsellors. The counsellor will take a fee and pay for the use of the services provided.

References

1   Pharmaceutical Services Negotiating Committee (2002) *Community Pharmacy: medicines management*. PSNC, London.
2   Department of Health (2002) *The NHS Plan*. The Stationery Office, London.
3   Report for the Community Pharmacy Research Consortium (March 2001) *Care at the Chemist: a question of access*. Available at www.rpsgb.org.uk/pdfs/minail.pdf
4   *Training Matters*. Communications International Group, London.
5   Li Wan Po A and G (1997) *OTC Medications: symptoms and treatments of common illnesses*. Blackwell Science, Oxford.
6   Porteous T *et al.* (2000) *Report to Scottish Pharmaceutical General Council*. Health Economic Research Unit, University of Aberdeen.
7   Department of Health (2000) *Pharmacy in the Future: implementing the NHS Plan*. The Stationery Office, London.
8   Roberts D (2002) *The Complete Dispenser* (4e). Communications International Group, London.

Chapter 12

So you only want a dispensary?

Sadly, you have read the book and come to fully understand just a little of what is involved in running a pharmacy and decided you want no part of it. Before throwing the book away in despair, do remember that you need not be at all involved in the running of the business. That, after all, is why you will employ that excellent superintendent pharmacist who will come to you with such glowing references. In any case, the pharmacists' professional body almost forbids you to dabble in the dispensary part of the business at all.

However, it is your business and if it is to thrive, then surely you and your partners as fellow directors must take more than a passing interest in what is going on. Not only that, it is your duty to give a lead to the pharmacist so that the business heads in the direction in which you all want it to go. But, there is no need to take a day-to-day interest in the nitty-gritty running of the firm.

Indeed, the RPS places full responsibility for that on your pharmacist's shoulders.

So, doctors, turn the pages back and start again. It cannot be all that difficult. After all, what have you been saying about pharmacists all these years?

Still unhappy or lacking in confidence and convinced that a pharmacist is a better man than you, Gunga Din?

On the other hand, maybe the regulations have yet to be changed and you want to get on with something in the meantime until you are able to open your own pharmacy. Fine, then let us talk about that quite different beast, a dispensary.

By definition a dispensary does not need a superintendent pharmacist and, therefore cannot sell P-only preparations. Under The Medicines Act, however, a doctor can sell any medicine to private patients or those with whom the doctor does not have an NHS contract to serve.

As with the pharmacy, there is a need to set up a separate dispensary company, as described in Chapter 5. Without that the GP is not able to sell medicines to NHS patients. The only exception to that rule is the dispensing doctor who has long been able to sell so-called 'blacklisted' medicines to dispensing patients and to them only.

Dispensing practices

As mentioned above, dispensing practices are, in the NHS, a special case. They may sell medicines to their dispensing patients, but only 'blacklisted' preparations.

Historically, this right was uniquely granted to dispensers and their patients by Kenneth Clarke when he was Health Secretary in 1984. Let there be no mistake, he did not do it willingly, but it was then that he introduced his 'Blacklist' of drugs and medicines which could no longer be prescribed and dispensed to NHS patients. That list is no longer the modest 100 or so that Mr Clarke banned, but has increased to over 3000, as set out in Part XVIII of *The Drug Tariff*.[1]

The original Dispensing Doctors' Association (DDA) was founded to fight this measure among others, the others being the newly imposed Clothier Regulations and the so-called 'clawback', discount redistribution scale.

When Mr Clarke proposed his restrictive list it was immediately seen that rural patients, unlike their urban cousins, could not pop down the road to buy the newly blacklisted medicines and would thus be at a disadvantage. Very quickly a national campaign was set up by the DDA with the fortunate result that dispensing doctors have, for 20 years, been permitted to sell anything that appears on the ever-increasing Section XVIIIA of *The Drug Tariff*.

For the record the Regulation says:

> A doctor may prescribe such items privately, though he may not charge for doing so and can sell such items only if he is a doctor entitled under the 1974 Regulations to dispense to a patient and then only to that patient in the course of treatment.

Why, oh, why do so few take advantage of that right, except when in trouble with a chemist?

Over the past 20 years several dispensing practices, not wishing to go so far as opening a pharmacy, have pre-empted a chemist's application by, perhaps, joining with village shopkeepers to open a dispensary. This would sell anything and everything, which the chemists would need to retail to supplement their NHS dispensing income. It has proved an efficient defence in a number of cases.

For some little while now I have been travelling the land, asking dispensing doctors why they do not take advantage of this right that they have been given. After all, it is illogical to provide prescription drugs for your patients and then force those same patients to make the trek into town to seek out a chemist for their OTC medicines.

Not only that, pharmacy and national politicians may well ask – Why should dispensing practice continue? If patients can visit the chemist for OTCs, why not for prescription medicines? After all, as you saw from the previous chapter, pharmacists are fearing that the converse question might be asked because doctors are being encouraged to provide full packs out of hours as part of their new contract.

Dispensing doctors who provide OTCs ensure that the practice has as full a record of the drugs used by their patients as is possible. This must be a major safety factor.

Dispensing doctors can:

- advertise the service in the practice leaflet and on the premises
- provide a price list in the surgery
- set their own prices – remember VAT
- set up an OTC repeat system, including safety checks
- check interactions of OTC with prescribed drugs.

Dispensing doctors who sell OTCs must:

- keep records, possibly on the computer with other data about the patient
- sell only to dispensing patients
- ensure that staff are well-trained – *see* Chapter 7
- not submit prescriptions to the pricing authority
- keep all private payments separate.

All that is very simple. Even the keeping of records because that will be done simultaneously with printing the label.

When talking about this I am occasionally asked – What, apart from political, are the benefits of selling OTCs? There are many. In fact, it is a win-win situation for everybody.

The benefits to patients include the following.

- Frequently an OTC is all they need.
- The availability of them at the surgery is very welcome.
- Ever since the abolition of Resale Price Maintenance (RPM) a few years ago, pricing has been advantageous for the dispensing practice.
- The record of the purchase is embedded on the computer for safety reasons.
- There is a one-stop service.

The benefits to the NHS include:

- there are major savings over the prescription of ethical drugs
- patients are more content
- doctors are more content
- GMS is improved with the extra income.

The benefits to doctors include:

- an increased income with less need for GMS2 'bean-counting'
- increased satisfaction at the improved, more complete service
- no 'discount clawback' on OTC sales
- increased safety as OTCs are cross-checked with prescribed items.

There are also benefits to pharmacists.

- They are partially relieved of a heavy burden.
- There is more time to devote to new roles.
- There is more time to devote to the NHS.

So, when you think about it, everybody gains if the dispensing doctor provides this very welcome service.

There are a number of points that should be carefully covered before starting OTC sales. The practice should check with the local authority if they are going into it in anything other than a small way. It may be that planning permission will be needed for change-of-use, but only if the business is expanded in a major fashion – as will be described below after this dispensing doctor section.

If the practice does not own its premises then, for similar reasons, it should check with the owners about any restrictive covenants, once again, only if the volume of sales is large. Mostly, it will not be.

Finally, again if sales are large, tell the PCO what you are doing. It should be of no interest to it, especially if you have a separate company (*see* Chapter 5) and have informed your patients of your interest in the business.

The dispensing doctor's dispensary's unique selling points

Briefly, this list will tell anyone why your patients should buy their OTCs from you rather than from anywhere else. They are compelling reasons. The dispensary:

- is in the right place at the right time – when the patient needs the medicines
- has a captive clientele ready to be advised
- has the patient's full medical and drug history on the same dispensary computer
- can always check the safety of the OTC with prescribed medicines
- is run efficiently and is familiar to the patient
- has qualified dispensary staff
- has customers who assume the doctors know which OTCs are effective
- has a full range of these effective products
- has free in-house publicity in the practice leaflet given to every patient
- is able to price competitively.

Stocking the OTC section

It is an unfortunate fact that many GSL products sold in pharmacies are completely ineffective except in a placebo fashion, or are duplicates of many others, or have never undergone any clinical trials to prove their effectiveness. So some order has to be sorted out of this.

Possibly the best way ahead is to involve the complete dispensary team in the debate as to what to include in the practice OTC formulary, then go about it by therapeutic class.

Right at the start, do bear in mind that it is not essential to carry large stocks of every product all year round. Many OTCs are seasonal and are heavily advertised by the makers well in advance. That excellent magazine *Chemist & Druggist* briefs its readers in good time about which TV and newspaper advertising campaigns will be happening. It is then that the dispensary should be stocked with the appropriate product, if the team approve of it.

There are additional ways of deciding what to include in the formulary. The team could:

- research patient choices by asking or using questionnaires
- read magazines, especially women's and health magazines
- visit pharmacies to see where other pharmacists are putting their money
- read pharmacy publications such as *Chemist & Druggist*
- take note when products begin to be advertised on television.

The final formulary should be reviewed seasonally, according to previous sales figures.

The next decision is to check with *The Drug Tariff* that the product is in Section XVIIIA, then decide in what quantity to buy and from whom.

Manufacturers and wholesalers may well set up discount deals, as for ethical prescription drugs. Ask. You will then need to set up deals and controls as for your dispensing ethicals. Ensure that they are just as watertight.

Following that, a price list should be drawn up. The recommended prices at which these products are on sale in pharmacies are listed in *The OTC Directory*[2], which every practice receives. The prices are also in the *Chemist & Druggist.*

It is highly unlikely, even with your limited overheads, that you will be able to undercut supermarket prices, but there may be little problem in beating the high-street chemist. Pay them a visit, or ask your spouses to, to find out.

In setting your prices, do remember that you will pay VAT, but not be able to reclaim it if you are not registered. A suggested formula could be: (Cost + VAT) + dispensing fee of, say 25%, and see how this compares with pharmacy prices.

The prepared price list is then displayed in the waiting room, the nurse's room and strategically around the premises. Every edition of the practice leaflet could carry an updated version as an insert together with all the previously listed advantages of buying from the dispensary, prominently including the safety features.

Preparing the dispensary for OTC sales

This is an additional service to NHS dispensing and it is possible that there will have to be some changes within the dispensary.

An early decision will be whether to have a separate OTC section or to mix them with the prescription drugs. Chapter 8 has given some indication about how pharmacy ethicals are 'shelved' and the inference is that OTC/GSLs should be completely separate as, even for ethicals, simple A–Z stocking will not be followed.

It is assumed that no additional premises will be needed, but will additional shelf and cupboard space have to be freed or devised?

Then there is the computer. Can it handle OTCs or will the software company need to be asked to modify it to do so? Will it be able to cross-check interactions with the patient's prescription medicines? Can it handle OTC records, labels and ordering? Will it be possible to bar-code and check items?

A not unimportant point is collecting payment for which a till will be needed in order to separate sales from NHS prescription charges. The till will aid the collection of accurate figures of private sales for the accountant, who will need accurate books.

Finally, can the dispensary counter be adapted, with, perhaps, a glass top, to display the goods on sale and will it be possible to make a feature of OTC packs and the price list in the waiting room?

Staff

No doubt, being an excellent dispensing practice, your staff will be well trained on prescription drugs, but will they need any additional training on simple ailments and OTC medications? *OTC Medications: symptoms and treatment of common*

illnesses[3] is an excellent starting point together with ongoing reading of *Chemist &
Druggist* and the *OTC Directory*. Publishers Communications International produce
an excellent free magazine called *Training Matters*[4] for pharmacy staff.

The staff should be encouraged to set up a cross-check and recall mechanism as
for prescribed drugs and to keep records on the computer.

It would also be commercially useful if the dispenser noted when and how
many patients requested an item not stocked. It may be sensible to add it to the
shelves if there is enough demand.

Finally, the ordering of OTCs could be designated to a separate staff member, if
there is one. One reputable supplier of OTC/GSL products is: Phoenix Healthcare;
0121 433 3030, although it must be said that I have found it extraordinarily difficult
to extract one of their recent and very extensive price lists out of them. Phoenix
offer attractive discounts. A case discount of 8%, a 2% discount for weekly delivery
and other promotional discounts are offered as they occur, that is, if you can get a
copy of their catalogue. They have 12 depots scattered around the UK.

Final suggestions and summary

To make the most of OTC sales, dispensary team meetings should be held
twice yearly to decide on the formulary. Early spring and late summer are perhaps
the best times, because it will be about then that the makers will be announcing
their forthcoming seasonal advertising campaigns – spring for antihistamines,
summer remedies and skincare; late summer for cough and cold preparations.
There is no point in missing these campaigns.

Make your decisions according to the effectiveness of the product. Many of
them were, after all, on the prescribing list recently before being added to the
3000-strong 'blacklist' of *The Drug Tariff*.

Squeeze the maximum discount from the manufacturers and wholesalers and
keep records of everything.

Strategy

As a dispensing practice you will be providing a new service and there is no point
in providing it in a half-hearted way. If you do not believe in it and nobody knows
about it you may as well not bother. So, in the words of the marketeers: *mean it
and market it!!*

I hope that covers the subject pretty well for dispensing, except to ask if you
want to expand into the sales of other retail products. If you do, then follow the
pattern of the non-dispensing practice described below.

Non-dispensing practices

Unfortunately for them non-dispensing practices are not permitted to sell
medicines, even blacklisted ones, to their NHS patients. The only way to get
around that is to follow the advice in Chapter 5 about setting up an independent
dispensary company or drug store but not a pharmacy.

Possibly the only reasons for doing that are entrepreneurism to supplement
the financial failures of the new GP contract or to pave the way for an eventual
pharmacy when the regulations become favourable. How much easier it should be

to slot in a pharmacy when the time came, if there was a separate business already up and running.

The drug store will be a profitable exercise if it sells a large enough range of products. It will not be as expensive to run as a pharmacy, because instead of an expensive superintendent pharmacist it may be managed by an experienced high-street retail manager or, perhaps preferably, by a qualified dispenser looking for greater responsibility.

The range of retail products that could be sold would follow the pattern earlier described for pharmacies (*see* Chapter 9) from the same suppliers. What a drug store cannot sell, without a pharmacist, are P-only medicines and POMs. Inevitably, the range of products and therefore the profitability, will hugely exceed that of the dispensing practice dispensary.

There are many matters to sort out in order to open your dispensary including:

• creating a separate dispensary/drug store company
• designing the premises, shelving, etc
• the alteration or creation of suitable space within your building or extending the premises
• recruiting trained staff for utmost safety
• abiding by the various regulations as in Chapter 4, except those relating to pharmacy
• deciding on appropriate GSL stock and retail goods
• determining any specialty – herbs, homoeopathicals, nutritions, etc.

Having a themed dispensary may add to its profitability and maybe it will be possible to employ, as manager, a complementary medicine specialist to whom patients could be referred from the general practice.

Dispensing practices need not be the only ones to benefit from retail sales. All the benefits mentioned for them will apply to an in-house dispensary in any primary care health centre. Once the business is set up, if the manager has been well chosen, there will be very little for the partners to do apart from the occasional board meeting. In fact, a really good manager may well be upset if the doctors have too great a hands-on approach.

The additional and major advantage will be that the future upgrading of the premises to a pharmacy will be simple, if that is kept in mind from the start at the design stage.

Conclusion

I hope that this book, apart from being a useful tool to the convinced, will have served to persuade medical colleagues that there is a great deal of satisfaction to be gained from owning a pharmacy – not to mention the additional income.

It has to be said that doctors who do embark on the path to pharmacy are going to meet some stiff opposition on the way. Most of it will be illogical and uninformed.

Over the years, many national politicians have swallowed the propaganda of the pharmacists and don't like the idea of doctors owning pharmacies, but there really is no logic in that attitude. If the service provided to the population by a given pharmacy is first class – and I hope that this book has encouraged that, through and through – then does it really matter who owns it? Of course not.

Nevertheless, it has been said by major politicians that doctors should be forbidden from pharmacy ownership. That knee-jerk response did not take heed of the Human Rights Act nor of the right of free trade of any legal company under whatever ownership.

Unfortunately, there is, in-built in all pharmacy politicians at the very least, a distrust of doctors. Over the years this has shown itself in their opposition and refusal to allow their colleagues to help in the training of dispensary staff for dispensing practices. Until recently the RPS refused to permit pharmacists to work in medical practices and so it went on.

Even now, some pharmacists are gearing themselves up to oppose the ownership of pharmacies by GPs, even though those pharmacies, as they legally must, will employ their colleagues as superintendent pharmacists. Indeed many may find that they are better paid by the owners of the in-house, one-stop primary care pharmacy, than by the high-street chain owners. There is little doubt that they will have the greater job satisfaction achieved, as in dispensing practice, by serving the same patients time and again. Patients are far more likely to become 'old friends' than ever would be the case in the high-street pharmacy.

Why, then, do the politicians oppose medically owned chemists? Is it because they fear job losses when the primary care pharmacy opens? But, as they say, as one door closes another opens. There is a shortage of pharmacists for the time being and any pharmacists who may lose their managership in the high street stand an excellent chance of finding better paid jobs in the health centre.

Is it because the chain owners have a large political clout? That may be so, because there is little doubt that the government inspired one-stop health centre will be found to be more convenient by patients and must affect high-street service more than a little.

Or is it because of the in-built bias of pharmacy against doctors as manifested by the multitude of dispensing disputes?

Whatever the reason is, it bears no foundation in common sense. There can be no answer to the fact that a well-run pharmacy is a well-run pharmacy.

I hope this book helps doctors to found and own just that sort of beast – a well-run pharmacy.

If you have any comments, please make contact either directly through the website www.countrydoctor.co.uk or through the publisher.

In addition, it may be possible to arrange a practice visit to help establish 'your own pharmacy'. Please contact me at davidroberts@doctors.org.uk or through the address on www.countrydoctor.co.uk.

References

1   Department of Health (Updated regularly) *The Drug Tariff*. Stationery Office, London.
2   Proprietary Association of Great Britain *OTC Directory 2003/2004. Treatments for Common Ailments*. Communications International Group, London.
3   Li Wan Po A and G (1997) *OTC Medications: symptoms and treatments of common illnesses*. Blackwell Science, Oxford.
4   *Training Matters* (monthly magazine). Communications International Group.

Appendix 1

Regulations and laws

Regulations

- NHS (General Medical & Pharmaceutical Services) Amendment (No. 2) Regulations 1987, No. 401 (Pharmacy Entry Regulations)
- NHS (Pharmaceutical Services) Regulation 1992 (Control of Entry Regulations)
- NHS (Pharmaceutical Services) Regulations 1992, No. 662 – Amendments to 1999
- NHS (General Medical & Pharmaceutical Services) Amendment Regulations 1983, No. 313 (The original Clothier rules)
- NHS (General Medical & Pharmaceutical Services) Amendment (No. 2) Regulations 1990, No. 1757 (Changes to Clothier)
- NHS (General Medical & Pharmaceutical Services) Amendment Regulations 1992, No. 662 (More changes to Clothier)

Laws

- The Asylum and Immigration Acts, 1996, 1999 and subsequent
- The Building Regulations 1991
- The Consumer Credit Act 1974
- The Consumer Protection Act 1987
- The Control of Substances Hazardous to Health Regulations 1988
- The Disability Discrimination Act 1995
- The Fire Precautions Act 1971
- The Fire Precautions (Workplace) Regulations 1997
- The General Product Safety Regulations 1994
- The Health & Safety (Young Persons) Regulations 1997
- The Intoxicating Substances (Supply) Act
- The Medicines Acts, 1968 and 1971
- The Misuse of Drugs Act 1971
- The Poisons Act 1972
- The Price Marking Order 1991
- The Race Relations Act 1976
- The Regulatory Reform Order 2004
- The Sale of Goods Act 1979
- The Sex Discrimination Acts, 1975 and 1984
- The Sunday Trading Act 1994
- The Supply of Goods and Services Act 1982
- The Trade Descriptions Act 1968

- The Working Time Directive 1998
- The Workplace (Health, Safety and Welfare) Regulations

All these may be obtained from The Stationery Office or referred to, online, through one of the search engines.

Appendix 2

Bibliography

- Barnes J, Anderson LA and Phillipson JD (2002) *Herbal Medicines: a guide for healthcare professionals*. Pharmaceutical Press, London.
- *British National Formulary*.
- *British Pharmacopoeia*.
- *Chemist & Druggist Directory*, published by CMP Data & Information Services, Tonbridge.
- *Chemist & Druggist Magazine*, published by CMP Data & Information Services, Tonbridge.
- Commons Health Committee (2003) *The Fifth Report of the Session 2002–03*. Stationery Office, London.
- Department of Health (updated regularly) *The Drug Tariff*. Stationery Office, London.
- Department of Health (2000) *The NHS Plan*. Stationery Office, London.
- *Guidance on Pharmacy Computer Systems*, published by Royal Pharmaceutical Society of Great Britain.
- Li Wan Po A and G (1997) *OTC Medications: symptoms and treatments of common illnesses*. Blackwell Science, Oxford.
- Medical Defence Union (1989) *Product Liability*. MDU, London.
- *Medicines Ethics and Practice: a guide for pharmacists*, No. 26 (July 2002), published by Royal Pharmaceutical Society of Great Britain.
- Merrills J and Fisher J (2001) *Pharmacy Law and Practice*. Blackwell Science, Oxford.
- *Pharmacy Business and Practice* (2003), published by National Pharmaceutical Association.
- *Pharmacy Magazine*, published by Communications International Group.
- *Primary Care Drug Dictionary*, published by Prescription Prescribing Authority.
- Proprietary Association of Great Britain. *OTC Directory 2003/2004. Treatments for Common Ailments*. Communications International Group, London.
- Roberts D (2002) *The Complete Dispenser* (4e). Communications International Group, London.
- *Sexual Orientation and the Workplace* (2003), published by ACAS.
- Spooner A (2004) *Quality in the New GP Contract: understanding, designing, planning, achieving*. Radcliffe Medical Press, Oxford.
- *Training Matters Magazine*, published by Communications International Group.

Appendix 3

List of contacts

- Association of Pharmacy Technicians, www.aptuk.org.uk
- *British Pharmacopoeia* Commission, Market Towers, 1 Nine Elms Lane, London, SW8 5NQ. Tel: 0207 720 9844
- Communications International Group, 309 Linen Hall, 162–168 Regent Street, London, W1R 5TB. Tel: 0207 434 1530
- Customs and Excise, New King's Beam House, 22 Upper Ground, London, SE4 9PJ. Tel: 0207 620 1313
- Department of Health:
    - Alexander Fleming House, Elephant & Castle, London, SE1 6BY. Tel: 0207 210 4850
    - Pharmaceutical Division, Portland Court, 158–176 Great Portland Street, London W1N 5TB
- Health & Safety Commission/Executive, Rose Court, 2 Southwark Bridge, London, SE1 9HS. Tel: 08701 545500
- Home Office, CS Division (Drugs Branch), Queen Anne's Gate, London, SW1H 9AT.
- National Health Service Confederation, Birmingham Research Park, Vincent, Birmingham, West Midlands, B15 2SQ. Tel: 0121 471 4444
- National Health Services (Northern Ireland) includes prescription pricing – 25–27 Adelaide Street, Belfast, BT2 8FH. Tel: 01232 324431
- National Pharmaceutical Association, 38–42 St Peter's Street, St Albans, Herts, AL1 3NP. Tel: 01727 832161
- Office of Fair Trading, Fleetbank House, 2–6 Salisbury Square, London, EC4Y 8JX.
- *Pharmaceutical Journal,* 1 Lambeth High Street, London, SE1 7JN. Tel: 0207 735 9141
- Pharmaceutical Services Negotiating Committee, 59 Buckingham Street, Aylesbury, Bucks, HP20 2PJ. Tel: 01296 432823
- Pharmaceutical Society of Northern Ireland, 73 University Street, Belfast, BT7 1HL
- Poisons Board, Home Office, 50 Queen Anne's Gate, London, SW1H 9AT
- Prescriptions Pricing Authority, Bridge House, 152 Pilgrim Street, Newcastle-upon-Tyne, NE1 6SN. Tel: 0191 232 5371
- Royal Pharmaceutical Society of Great Britain, 1 Lambeth High Street, London, SE1 7JN. Tel: 0207 735 9141
- Scottish Pharmaceutical Federation, 135 Buchanan Street, Glasgow, G1 2JA. Tel: 0141 221 1235
- Secretary of State for Health, Richmond House, 79 Whitehall, London SW1A 2NS. Tel: 0207 236 1189

- Society of Apothecaries, Apothecaries Hall, Blackfriars Lane, London, EC4V 6EJ. Tel: 0207 236 1189
- Stationery Office, 51 Nine Elms Lane, London, SW8 5DR
- Ulster Chemists Association, 73 University Street, Belfast, BT7 1HL. Tel: 01232 320787
- Welsh Pricing Committee, Prescription Pricing Office, Caradog House, 1–6 St Andrew's Place, Cardiff, CF1 3PY. Tel: 01222 372611/5

Appendix 4

List of websites

- Advisory Conciliation and Arbitration Service www.acas.org.uk
- Association of Pharmacy Technicians www.aptuk.org
- Association of Security Consultants www.securityconsultants.org.uk
- *Bandolier* www.jr2.ox.ac.uk/bandolier
- *British Medical Journal* www.bmj.com
- *British National Formulary* www.bnf.org
- *British Pharmacopoeia* Commission www.pharmacopoeia.org.uk
- *Chemist & Druggist Magazine* www.dotpharmacy.com
- Community pharmacy www.medicinesmanagement.org.uk
- Community pharmacy www.managingmedicines.com
- Companies House www.companieshouse.gov.uk
- *Country Doctor* magazine www.countrydoctor.co.uk
- Customs & Excise www.hmce.gov.uk
- Department of Health Northern Ireland: www.dhsni.gov.uk
- Department of Health Scotland www.scotland.gov.uk
- Department of Health Wales www.wales.gov.uk
- Department of Health www.doh.gov.uk
- Dot Pharmacy www.dotpharmacy.com
- Electronic Medicines Compendium www.emc.vhn.net
- Em Recruitment www.emrecruitment.co.uk
- Enigma Health plc www.enigmahealth.com
- Health & Safety Commission www.hse.gov.uk
- Health news www.health-news.co.uk
- Home Office www.homeoffice.gov.uk
- Inland Revenue www.inlandrevenue.gov.uk
- *Lancet* www.thelancet.com
- Medicines Control Agency www.mca.gov.uk
- Medicines Information Service www.druginfozone.org
- Medline–American Library of Medicine www.medscape.com
- *Merck Manual* www.merck.com/pubs
- National Approved Council for Security Systems www.nacoss.org
- National electronic Library for Health www.nelh.nhs.uk
- National Pharmaceutical Association www.npa.co.uk
- National Prescribing Centre www.npc.co.uk
- National Security Inspectorate www.nsi.org.uk
- Office of Fair Trading www.oft.gov.uk
- *Pharmaceutical Journal* www.pharmj.com
- Pharmaceutical Services Negotiating Committee www.psnc.org.uk/database

- Pharmacy in the future www.rpsgb.org.uk/nhsplan/index
- Implementing the NHS Plan www.doh.gov.uk/pharmacyfuture
- Pharmacy Locums UK www.pharmacylocumsuk.com
- Pharmacy online www.priory.com/pharmol
- Pharmacy Relief Staff Agency www.pharmacyrelief.co.uk
- Prescription Pricing Authority www.ppa.org.uk
- Prescription Pricing Authority www.ppa.org.uk
- *Primary Care Drug Dictionary* www.ppa.org.uk/systems/pcdd_intro.htm
- Primary Care Pharmacists Association www.pcpa.org.uk
- Proprietary Association of Great Britain www.pagb.co.uk
- Reed Health Professionals www.reedhealth.co.uk
- Royal Pharmaceutical Society www.rspgb.org.uk
- Scottish Pharmaceutical Federation www.rpsgb.org/scotland
- Security Systems and Alarms Inspection Board www.ssaib.co.uk
- Society of Apothecaries www.apothecaries.org.uk
- Stationery Office www.tso.gov.uk
- UK Medicines Information www.ukmi.nhs.uk

Index

Page numbers in *italics* refer to tables or figures.